A Deaf Adult Speaks Out

Leo M. Jacobs

Second Edition, Revised and Expanded

Gallaudet College Press

Published by the Gallaudet College Press
Kendall Green, Washington, D.C. 20002

Library of Congress Catalog Card
Number 80-83505

Gallaudet College is an equal opportunity employer/educational institution. Programs and services offered by Gallaudet College receive substantial financial support from the Department of Education.

ISBN 0-913580-63-5

Dedication

This literary effort is dedicated to the memory of my late wife, Dorothy, and to my daughters, Sheila and Lisa, for their encouragement and their willingness to endure my long absence from home and hearth which made possible my initial effort in writing this book.

Acknowledgements

To the Board of Directors of Gallaudet College, President Edward C. Merrill, Jr., of Gallaudet College, and the Powrie V. Doctor Chair Committee, sincere appreciation is extended for their support and encouragement.

To Dr. McCay Vernon, Dr. Gilbert L. Delgado, Dr. Norman Tully, and Dr. Mervin D. Garretson, the writer is very grateful for their willingness to spare some of their valuable time to review the draft and offer constructive suggestions and advice. Sincere thanks are also due Dr. Garretson for his review of the material for the revision.

To Ms. Lolly Gilbert, the writer also wishes to extend his sincere thanks for her invaluable services in the editing of the original manuscript and to Ms. Barbara Brissenden and Dr. Kathleen Callaway for their editing of the revised edition.

To others, including the staff of the Edward Miner Gallaudet Memorial Library, this opportunity is taken to express gratitude for their willing assistance and rendering of information.

About the Author

Frequently society is made aware of the problems and status of a minority or a group of people who deviate from the so-called mainstream. This awareness is usually articulated and/or interpreted by a sociologist or other professional person. Some of these writers do a masterful job of research, of living close to the setting, of getting data directly from the people concerned. Notwithstanding their professional skills, there is one vital dimension missing—that is, having actually *lived* the experience. Even living the experience must be qualified in terms of length of time, whether one is born into it, or whether it evolved, and also the degree or, if you will, the level within the setting where the experience occurs. Seldom does the voice of the "grassroots" come directly from the grassroots. The obvious reason is the lack of expressive skills to tell the story. Fortunately, from time to time, society hears from someone who has lived the experience and can tell the story.

Such a person is Leo M. Jacobs. When he was chosen from a group of very well-qualified applicants to be the first Professor of the Powrie V. Doctor Chair, the winning phrase was: "Leo is a deaf person—head to toe." It was time the hearing and the deafened and the world in general should hear from such a person. Jacobs was born deaf. His parents and his brother are deaf. His wife, who is deceased, was deaf. Leo has one deaf and one hearing child. He has, in a very real sense, grown up and lived in the silent world of a deaf society. He has succeeded in a "hearing world" but identifies and relates extremely well with every stratum of deaf society.

After completing his schooling at the California School for the Deaf, Berkeley, Leo matriculated at Gallaudet College where he received a B.A. degree in 1938. He qualified and passed the entrance examination for Gallaudet at the age of 14. After working as a boys' counselor for 9 years at his *alma mater* in Berkeley, he became a teacher in the high school department in 1947. During this time Leo developed a ''Practical Language'' course of study still in use at Berkeley and quite a few other schools. In 1957 he earned a master's degree at San Francisco State College.

Leo's professional awareness is demonstrated by his participation in four summer institutes in the areas of mathematics. (He is a master math teacher.) He is a member of the Convention of American Instructors of the Deaf, the Registry of Interpreters for the Deaf and the California State Employees' Association. His dedication to serving deaf people is manifest by his work and the offices held in organizations such as the Deaf Counseling, Advocacy, and Referral Agency, formerly the East Bay Counseling and Referral Agency for the Deaf (a truly effective service for deaf people operated by deaf people), National Association of the Deaf, Gallaudet College Alumni Association, National Fraternal Society of the Deaf, California Home for the Aged Deaf, and numerous others. He has presented papers on topics relating to the socio-economic and social behavior of the deaf adult, the need for strong central organization of deaf people, interpreters, and various academic topics.

I have had the personal good fortune to have known Leo Jacobs since 1958. I have known him as a fellow teacher of deaf adults, as an administrator in a high school for the deaf, and as a friend. Leo has been an ''education'' for me. Directly and indirectly, he provided me insights to feeling deafness and, more importantly, to respecting and accepting deaf persons as they are, not as we wish to make them. The Jacobs family is a delight—happy, outgoing, communicating, and healthy in every way. This, too, tells its own story. Using today's parlance, Jacobs is eminently qualified to know from whence it came, to put it all together, and to say it like it is.

Gilbert L. Delgado, Ph.D.
Assistant Vice President
for Academic Affairs, and
Dean, Graduate School
Gallaudet College

Foreword

The Gallaudet College Board of Directors established the Powrie Vaux Doctor Chair of Deaf Studies in the spring of 1972. This Chair was established in memory of Professor Powrie Vaux Doctor, a member of the Gallaudet College faculty for 43 years, who died in Paris in the summer of 1971 while attending meetings of the World Federation of the Deaf. At the time of his death, Dr. Doctor was serving Gallaudet as a professor of government, chairman of the Department of Government, and acting dean of the Graduate School.

A committee of Gallaudet alumni, faculty, student, and administration representatives selects an appointee to the Chair for each academic year. Such appointments are reserved for resident teacher-scholars in the field of deaf education (or educational programs for deaf students) who show potential for or have made significant contributions to the field.

I had the honor of being the first recipient of the Chair for the academic year 1972-1973. I saw, in the offer of the Doctor Chair, a chance to "tell it like it is" about the world of deaf adults—which has been my world, too.

As a person, born deaf, who has also spent 42 years working with deaf children and interacting with the adult deaf community as a volunteer worker and leader, I have seen many failures and met comparatively few successes in the traditional educational methods used with deaf persons.

The average deaf child usually has hearing parents who are unable to communicate with him. When I was younger, I was distressed by the seeming inevitability of inadequate education for such children. But, as I grew older and more aware, my feelings turned to disgust and indignation, because I began to realize that the inadquacies in the education of deaf children were not inevitable. Instead, they were being preserved by hearing educators who seemed to know too little about the end-products of their system.

What follows may not possess the degree of objectivity nor the pedantry that might normally characterize such a contribution. Instead, concern, anger, and genuine feeling for the shortchanging that deaf people have been receiving are predominant.

Leo M. Jacobs

Contents

1 Introduction

In order for people unacquainted with deafness* and its problems to know and understand deaf people, they should first become familiar with certain factors which contribute to the personal development of deaf adults. These include environment, etiology of hearing loss, education, and training. But, the most important factor of all is the persons: parents, teachers, supervisors at work, friends and relatives, and possibly clergy, social workers, rehabilitation personnel, or counselors who mold the deaf person's total development.

Since we live in a society in which hearing people are dominant, these responsible people, with a few exceptions, are hearing. The sad truth is that comparatively few of these hearing persons have either the intimate experience with deafness or the empathy for deaf people which is necessary before they can really become effective. Whatever help or advice they offer the deaf persons coming under their spheres of authority or influence is dispensed out of only a vicarious understanding of deafness. This understanding is not fully internalized and felt.

The personal life experience which has contributed to this manuscript is revelant. I am a deaf adult who has been deaf since birth; a deaf child of deaf parents who married a deaf woman; a deaf parent of a deaf child and a hearing child; a dormitory counselor of deaf boys for nine years; a teacher of high school age deaf children for 28 years; a coordinator of continuing and community education, informally for three years, and formally for four years; and an acquaintance or a personal friend of the deaf friends of my parents, the deaf friends of my older deaf brother, my deaf schoolmates from my school and

*See Glossary, p. 138.

college years, my former deaf students and their friends, deaf adults from not only my local community but also the national community of the deaf, my colleagues in the field of deafness—both deaf and hearing, and hearing parents, hearing workers in the field of deafness, and interested hearing friends of the deaf, in both my professional and civic activities.

My own life experience has involved intimate exposure to a large segment of the adult deaf population, creating an awareness of the many and varied ways in which deaf people have been repressed, restrained, and frustrated in their search for an adequate education and an equal opportunity for a meaningful life. I have seen thousands of deaf adults who have been stopped drastically short of their full potential by unthinking, presumptuous, sometimes selfish, or even plainly ignorant, people* who happened to have had a hand in these deaf adults' development.

Therefore, it is my hope to demonstrate in this book that the deaf have had to contend with handicaps beyond that of their loss of hearing, and that these additional obstructions have been much more significant than their deafness in the general retardation of their development.

---

*This is not meant to be a sweeping indictment of hearing professionals working with deaf persons, but rather that of hearing persons possessing traditional attitudes toward deafness. There has always been a small group of hearing educators who have been real friends to deaf people. Thus, hearing people in the field of deafness might be categorized in two different groups.

The first and traditional group seems to regard the handicap first, and deaf persons as individuals second. Thus, their efforts have been mainly to "conquer" deafness by concentrating on the normalizing of deaf youngsters so that they can "speak and listen" like hearing children, to the cost of their many other needs. They seem to be much more clinical and standoffish in their attitude, and to regard deaf people more like case studies than as human beings.

The second group has an entirely different attitude; they are more interested in deaf persons as individuals in their own right than in their deafness. They socialize much more often with deaf people, and thereby gain empathy that the first group does not seem to possess. Modern emphasis on total communication and realistic practicum methods, which include interaction not only with deaf children but also with local deaf communities, is producing an increasing number of hearing professionals in the second category, for which we are grateful.

2 What Deafness Means

Most people are familiar with the dictionary definition of deafness, which is the absence of hearing. However, this is an oversimplification since the deprivation of one's hearing can vary both in its degree and kind.

Let us consider, in theory, a human being in the full possession of health, mind, and faculties with a single exception: the ability to hear. What does this loss of one faculty do to a person who is otherwise perfectly "normal"?

Such a question defies a simple answer, for so many factors are involved. Perhaps the first and most important factor that comes to mind is when this loss occurred. There is a big difference between an onset of deafness at birth and at the age of 25.

Onset of Deafness

The sense of hearing serves as one of our main channels for the input of information. The adult who loses the ability to hear has had the full benefit of that sense during development from untutored infant to adult. This person has grown up learning normal language ability, oral* skills, and those requisite skills needed for a satisfactory standard of living. But, a child who was born deaf is an entirely different proposition. This child has had a strike called against him/her right from birth. A deaf child's sense of hearing can give only imperfect or distorted input of information so the youngster will have to acquire living skills through other channels of communication.†

*See Glossary, p. 139.
†See Glossary, p. 138.

Any competent educator in the field of deafness knows that the difference of even one or two years in the age of the onset of deafness can make a noticeable difference in a person's development. But, average people who are in full possession of their hearing have no concept at all of the large part that the sense of hearing plays in their own development, nor even in their communication with the outside world. They have taken this sense so much for granted that they have never once thought of how it would be without the ability to hear.

This excerpt from *In This Sign,* Joanne Greenberg's perceptive novel on deafness, may serve to clarify what I am driving at.

> Mrs. Anglin had two cups and saucers and she picked up the coffeepot with her free hand and began to move forward. Janice had stopped and half-turned and Mrs. Anglin cried, "Watch out—this is still hot!" The movement of Janice's arm did not stop. Mrs. Anglin found herself blocked by the table; she couldn't move back. Janice's arm was still moving around with her turning. "Get back, look out, you'll get burned!"
>
> Margaret, coming from the kitchen, heard her mother-in-law cry out and looked up too late to see anything but her expression of irritation giving way to one of fascinated horror. Janice's upper arm was stopped firmly against the hot side of the coffeepot. With a strangle-sound she pulled away violently and cutlery scattered from the plate she was still holding. The reflex movement had turned her around and she was facing Mrs. Anglin with a wounded vulnerable expression, like a child beaten for no reason. She touched the arm gingerly. The flesh had gone white and then red and even now an angry red blotch was coming out plainly. Mrs. Anglin's voice sounded pettish. She felt guilty and was also perhaps at the end of her patience with the evening.
>
> "I told you . . . I called out and you—well, you just *stood* there!" Her face had lost all its softness again. "Why didn't you get out of the way? I told you—"
>
> Margaret had come around to Mrs. Anglin's side and was Signing gently to Janice: "She told you to get out of the way, but you didn't hear her." Janice opened a slow, half-frightened smile, and said in her tiny Sign, "I'm sorry—it's not a bad burn. It only startled me."

Mrs. Anglin looked around in wonder and then her hand came up to her face. "How could I have done that? You told me she was deaf—that both your parents were deaf. I saw your father making the Signs but somehow, somehow I didn't believe—I didn't really believe it could be. Is it possible, really possible that a person can not hear at all? (pp. 178-179)

Dr. Edna Simon Levine also points this out beautifully in her book *The Psychology of Deafness:*

The unimpaired counterpart of deafness is hearing. And it happens that the values of hearing in human experience are generally as little recognized and as difficult to grasp as the implications of deafness. Both are intangible functions that operate through unseen structures. Neither provides visual aids to understanding.

Further, to hear is as natural and effortless an occurrence as it is invisible. Man would as soon ask himself how breathing keeps him physically alive as how hearing keeps him psychologically alive. He simply does not think of it at all. As for the handicaps of auditory defect, they are equally hidden from view. They do not "show, the way a distorted limb or a missing finger or blinded eyes 'show.' " The sufferer " 'limps' only socially, 'fumbles' only psychologically, 'stumbles' only vocationally." Crippling takes place in ways that are not readily observed, and because of this the implications of auditory handicaps are not easy to identify.

To obtain the "feel" of deafness, therefore, is a difficult assignment for one who hears. (pp. 17-18)

Average hearing people, for the most part, are so used to watching the other party's face and lips while talking that these people are unaware that they are not really watching but rather listening to the speaker. Hence, hearing people are receptive to the often implied concept that lipreading can be a complete form of communication—that deaf persons can learn to read lips as well as hearing people hear. Nothing is further from the truth.

The same people also learned to speak without any effort. Again, these hearing persons are not conscious of the role hearing plays in acquisition of speech; they are often unaware that hearing enables one to listen to and to monitor one's own speech. It is because they can hear that they are able to develop normal speech effortlessly. Thus, it is often difficult for them to comprehend that speech is either very difficult or impossible for a hearing impaired* individual to develop.

However, once the readers are able to grasp these concepts of deafness, they should be able to understand how even an additional year or two with full possession of hearing can mean much toward a more optimum development of a child who may be deafened later, for the child would be in possession of an appreciably greater amount of knowledge, information, and perception at the time of the loss of hearing.

Degree of Hearing Loss

Another factor which must be reckoned with is the degree of hearing loss, because it is not often that a person is totally deaf. Most deaf persons can hear certain sounds, i.e., they have what is called residual hearing.

In their book *They Grow in Silence,* Drs. Eugene Mindel and McCay Vernon refer to residual hearing in the following way:

> Residual hearing is a catchall phrase referring to the hearing available after damage to the auditory mechanism has already occurred. It can refer to useless sensitivity to low-pitched sounds, or to functionally useful remnants of hearing in the higher pitched ranges. Unless the amount and extent of residual hearing is defined, this information, given to parents, can create an unrealistic fantasy that the child will develop normal speech and language—that he will no longer be deaf.
>
> Speech consists of a relatively narrow range of pitches, mostly between 300 and 4000 cycles per second. The value of residual hearing depends, in part, upon a combination of loudness and pitch—the loudness required before the sound can be heard by the child and the pitch ranges (cycles per second) the child can hear. Therefore, the potential for learning speech through residual hearing may be nonexistent or it may be excellent. Interpretations con-

*See Glossary, p. 138.

cerning the significance of residual hearing in relation to speech
and language should be given conservatively. Unfortunately they
are generally too optimistic.

Audiologists have encountered persons who have normal hearing only at the higher frequency ranges—2000 to 4000 cycles per
second. With this preservation of hearing, these rare individuals
have been able to develop normal language and speech. This is apparently because they can perceive consonant sounds accurately.
Consonants carry the information of speech, and are heard as high
frequency sounds. Unfortunately, most deaf and hard of hearing
children have the least hearing in these high frequency ranges.
(pp. 34-35)

Then, the *amount* of loss should be considered, for it is obvious, even to the layman, that the greater the amount of loss,
the less likely it is for a person to hear well, even if one's hearing is amplified.

Two interesting definitions of deafness are relevant to this.
In 1937 the Convention of American Instructors of the Deaf
adopted a resolution revising the nomenclature used in the field
of deafness:

> **The deaf:** those in whom the sense of hearing is non-
> functional for the ordinary purposes of life. This general
> group is made up of two distinct classes based entirely
> on the time of the loss of hearing: (a) the congenitally
> deaf—those who were born deaf; (b) the adventitiously
> deaf—those who were born with normal hearing, but in
> whom the sense of hearing is non-functional later
> through illness or accident.
>
> **The hard of hearing*:** those in whom the sense of
> hearing, although defective, is functional with or with-
> out a hearing aid.

Dr. Jerome Schein, while at the Office of Demographic
Studies at Gallaudet College, devised the following scale of

*See Glossary, p. 138.

deafness, which helps to distinguish between its different degrees:

Scale of Deafness

1. I can hear loud noises.
2. I can usually tell one loud noise from another.
3. I can usually tell the sound of speech from other sounds.
4. I can usually HEAR AND UNDERSTAND a few words if I can see the speaker's face and lips.
5. I can usually HEAR AND UNDERSTAND a few words without seeing the speaker's face and lips.
6. I can usually HEAR AND UNDERSTAND most of the things a person says to me if I can see his face and lips.
7. I can usually HEAR AND UNDERSTAND most of the things a person says to me without seeing his face and lips.
8. I can usually HEAR AND UNDERSTAND a discussion between several people without seeing their faces and lips.
9. I can usually HEAR AND UNDERSTAND telephone conversations with a special telephone or amplifier.
10. I can usually HEAR AND UNDERSTAND a telephone conversation on any telephone.

The graded responses on this scale are items 1, 2, 3, 5, and 7. The items, in that order, have a logical validity in that it is logical that a person who would answer "No" to item 1 would then answer "No" to all the following items. Assigning one point for every "Yes" answer, those who obtain scores of less than 5 most typically have been found to have hearing losses of 70 decibels or more. From extensive testing conducted at Gallaudet College in Washington, D.C., it is apparent that persons are able to give a reasonably accurate estimate of their hearing status.

The Real Handicap of Deafness

Although my main topic is deaf adults who are otherwise normal, three more notable points about deafness need mention.

First, when a child becomes deaf from an outside cause, such as illness or accident during the pregnancy of the mother or after his birth, it is not uncommon that some other handicap accompanies the deafness.

Therefore, statistics show a higher incidence of additional handicaps among the deaf than among the general public. As modern medicine creates a higher rate of survival among such afflicted children, it is thereby turning out more and more deaf children who need special programs and attention. The present schools and programs for deaf children are ill-prepared to handle these children with additional and special problems. But, increasing concern is being shown for these multihandicapped deaf children and pressure is being built up now to create special programs or institutions for them, such as the special units at both state schools for the deaf in California.

Secondly, another fact to consider is that the greatest handicapping effect of deafness is the cutting off of normal vocal communication. This point can not be emphasized too strongly, for this fact alone is responsible for numerous of the problems which accompany deafness. These problems appear because too many people misinterpret the meaning of communication, and fail to comprehend the consequences of the lack of a full and complete channel through which language can be sent into a deaf child.

Consider a child who is normal in every way except for his deafness. He was born a bundle of pulsating humanity, with every bone, muscle, and nerve intact and ready to function, except for a lesion in the auditory pathway. There is nothing wrong with his voice box, and this should quickly become ap-

parent when the deaf infant starts to register anger when
frustrated or ignored. Every time his mother kisses the pair of
pink, delicate ears they are to all appearances normal. His
brain is in perfect working order, for his parents and pediatri-
cian can see him developing in almost every aspect: learning
how to coordinate his eyes so that he can see clearly; reaching
out his tiny hands until he learns to grasp objects; squirming
until he learns how to turn over; and so forth.

Because the child is not receiving sound impulses, his
behavior begins to deviate; unnoticeably at first. Then, as the
differences become more pronounced, the parents are puzzled
and uneasy. Perhaps the first thing which is usually suspected
is the baby's mind, for when behavior aberration is noticed,
mental retardation is usually thought of first. Most pediatri-
cians are not familiar with the effects of deafness on an infant
and often fail to make the diagnosis early.

When deafness is finally diagnosed, hearing parents who are
unfamiliar with deafness are usually panic-stricken. Their first
thought is to "normalize" the child, to make him behave as
much like a child with perfect hearing as possible. Therefore,
they subscribe readily to the philosophy of oralism.* That a
deaf child can eventually speak and "hear" visible speech is
quite a heady thing for anxious hearing parents who are otherwise unacquainted with the many and varied problems of
deafness.

The experiences of Lee Katz, the mother of a deaf girl, as
graphically described in an article in *The Deaf American* only illustrate what countless thousands of hearing parents who knew
nothing about deafness went through, or are now going
through, so that they would not fail their deaf children:

> Since we'd discovered Liz's deafness when she was a little over a
> year old, we'd embarked on teaching her speech and lipreading
> with such intensity that the beautiful levity of life was a scarcity.

*See Glossary, p. 139.

We had such a mental set—such an immovable focus on the goal of speech and lipreading skills—there was room for precious little of anything else. The day of the tongue-thrusting (at her teacher) marked a slow beginning to the search for a more natural, healthy way by which to communicate. We had no intentions of giving up speech and lipreading, but we felt deeply that this young child was due a great deal more.

Up to this time we had depended solely on the literature and advice of people and organizations embracing complete oralism as the means to educate and fulfill the life of a deaf child. These sources were always entirely available, in person and through the mails. Like the eager insurance lawyer at the scene of the accident, handing out his card to a prospective client, they were always there first. Just as importantly, they said and wrote everything we hearing parents ever wanted to hear: Through speech and lipreading there would be complete integration into the hearing world. What wasn't said, among many other things, was that speech and lipreading skills are only a part of what a human being requires, and that supplemental methods of education and communication are imperative. Lizabeth's rebellion at her teacher that day began to bring home this kind of thinking. (p. 35)

The comments of Mary Jane Rhodes, the mother of a deaf boy, in her column in *The Deaf American,* brings us further insight into what the hearing parents of a deaf child have to face:

It is very difficult for hearing parents of deaf children to accept the fact that their baby cannot hear. With no understanding of the handicap they are at a loss to know what to do to help their son or daughter who is deaf. Mothers and fathers want to do what is best for their deaf youngster, but they are confused and uncertain as to what their child needs.

It hurts, but parents can accept and understand that their child cannot hear the birds sing and the wind blow. They can accept the knowledge that their baby won't hear bells ring or the sound of rain on the window. What they cannot accept or understand is that they can't communicate with this important member of their family . . . I have seen cases where hearing parents have rejected their deaf child. Virtually every week there is a new story to be told of how deaf boys and girls are facing problems because they cannot communicate with their parents. It is almost always the parents who are blamed for not accepting and adjusting to their deaf child's handicap. But how can we blame the parents, when they have never truly been told and shown how to communicate with their child? (p. 26)

Those parents may find the following contrasting side of the picture of deafness interesting.

Roger M. Falberg described his experience in his column, "Sifting the Sands," in *The Silent Worker* in 1957 as follows:

> I was the "great experiment," the deaf child "restored" to the hearing world attending public schools . . . Loneliness.
>
> That's all it ever was, and all it will be to me—stark, staring, tearing loneliness . . . I doubt if I need to explain here what I mean by loneliness. Surely everyone knows how cruel children can be to the child who is "different" in some way or another. They jeer at the child who is wealthy, sneer at the poor boy's clothes and throw mud at the sissies. Then, in time, the rich boy learns democracy, and pauper betters himself, and the coward rears up and fights back. But the deaf child never learns to hear.

My experience was very different from Falberg's and from that of most deaf children.

I was born deaf of deaf parents who had an older deaf son. Therefore, my family was entirely deaf, and we lived in a world of our own, where manual communication was the order of the day. I grew up in a loving atmosphere and never knew any deprivation of communication; my parents knew my wants, and I knew just how far I could go without bringing their wrath down on my head. The conversation was full and interesting at the dinner table. I learned all the facts of life at appropriate times. I attended a residential school as a day pupil. My only communication difficulties arose when I began doing business with the outside world, but I thought nothing about them because I had observed my parents' methods of overcoming those barriers. I merely followed the same road—that of employing a pad and pencil to convey my wishes, and attempting to read lips at first, then offering the pad and pencil to the other party if I failed to understand him.

For a deaf infant to develop normally from the child to the adult who knows that he is loved and who is inspired to utilize his mind and talents to the utmost, total communication* is needed; for if the child only perceives limited or no communication, then his brain and personality lie fallow, and are likely to become incapacitated due to lack of use.

Thus, my third point is that the most crippling effect of deafness is the fact that many parents and educators fail to realize the critical need for "full communication." This means an open, facile communication where meaningful responses are the rule, not mere monosyllabic utterances such as "Yes," "No," "Mommy," etc.

*See Glossary, p. 139.

3 What Communication Really Is

The peoples of the world, no matter what their cultures and beliefs, will readily identify communication with hearing and speech. This is not surprising since the primary tools of communication throughout the known world are hearing and speech.

However, communication is not necessarily limited to hearing and speech. The *Webster's New World Dictionary* succinctly defines communication as "a transmitting; a giving, or giving and receiving, of information, signals, or messages by talk, gestures, writing, etc." The important aspect of the dictionary definition of communication is *the transmittal of information.*

Parents and educators working with deaf children frequently fail to understand and appreciate the fact that a child's deafness precludes normal reception of sound impulses, and that visible speech, even under the best possible conditions permits only a small part of the messages to be understood.

Mindel and Vernon have this to say about comprehension of lipreading in *They Grow in Silence:*

> Edgar Lowell's 1957, 1958, and 1959 studies conducted by the Tracy Clinic illustrated the problems inherent in speech reading. Nondeaf college sophomores who had never studied speech reading were more successful at it than deaf persons to whom it had been taught throughout most of their school careers. The better performance by the nondeaf sophomores derived from their normal language base (phonetic, semantic, and syntactic), enabling them to determine by guessing the words they could not speech read. It is helpful to remember that 40 to 60 percent of English sounds are monophonous: their formation on the lips is identical to that of other sounds. A person without an adequate language base to fill in the gaps understands very little. In fact, even the best speechreaders in a one-to-one situation were found to understand

only 26 percent of what was said. Many bright deaf individuals
grasp less than five percent. (p. 26)

Therefore, when you consider untrained and undisciplined
deaf infants or small children, it seems to approach the
ridiculous if their parents attempt to communicate by talking,
talking, and talking to them. For, to many of those without
normal hearing, including myself, the lip movements of people
talking convey very little meaning. Much of the time we see
them only as flapping lips.

It is possible for a hearing person to get a little of this sensa-
tion by sitting down before the television set and then turning
out all the sound. Do this just before an episode starts, and then
try following the thread of the plot throughout the story. It
takes quite a bit of ingenuity and guesswork to do it satisfac-
torily. After this little test, it will give the viewer a welcome and
comfortable feeling to be able to tune in the sound again and
enjoy the television. This would be a good time to pause and
reflect that a deaf person cannot and will not ever be able to
tune in any sound except, perhaps, for some static. Moreover,
the deaf person most likely does not have the background
knowledge of language patterns which aid in lipreading that the
average hearing viewer has.

This is not meant to depreciate the real value of training in
speech and speech reading; they have their rightful place in an
educational program for deaf children. Yet, the crux of the
matter is to get the needed information through to infants and
small children who are deaf. Educators have reiterated that the
ripest time to start training and educating children is the years
between birth and five years of age.

Therefore, the prime concern of the parents of little deaf
children should be to get the necessary information through to
them before their active little minds are starved from a dearth
of incoming data, and possibly become too incapacitated to accept a normal amount of input.

Thomas Goulder in the *Guest Lecturer Series,* 1971, at the
North Carolina School for the Deaf emphasized the importance
of having familial communication:

> Communication courses for parents must begin at the earliest
> stages of development so that the deaf child becomes a real person
> within the family and shares in all the joys and sorrows of family.
> (pp. 133-134)

The parents of little deaf children should let their love and
concern for the best welfare of their children override any pride
or prejudice they may possess, and start using any method of
communication that will readily reach the youngsters' minds,
and elicit response from them. They should not be ashamed to
use exaggerated gestures to implement their speech although
they would be doing their children a big favor if they would
learn some formal signs* beforehand. Homemade gestures are
equivalent to baby talk, and are therefore worthless outside the
immediate family, while formal signs can be carried over to
other situations. Other good ancillary methods would be using
facial expressions and/or body movements, and drawing pictures. There have been some questions about using fingerspell-
ing† alone with very little children, for they may not be ready
to read the small movements until approximately the same
time that they are ready to read the printed word.

If small children are too immature to look at and distinguish
small printed letters of the alphabet in order to develop their
reading skills, then how can they read the hard-to-distinguish
lip movements, especially if they have very few concepts
already established in their minds?

To repeat, I am not against the employment of speech-reading
and lipreading; in fact, no deaf adults are against their use.
Total communication (TC) is supported by the overwhelming

*See Glossary, p. 139.
†See Glossary, p. 138.

majority of deaf adults, and is the official policy of the National Association of the Deaf. Total communication includes the use of speech and lipreading along with the use of homemade gestures, facial expressions, body movements, formal signs, fingerspelling, writing, illustrating, amplification devices, and whatever other methods will reach deaf children.

However, our priorities differ from those of hearing parents and educators who champion the oral method. We consider the training in oral methods of communication to be a matter of convenience, not a matter of life or death. We feel they should take a back seat to the all-important mission of communicating fully with the children so that we are sure they are getting an adequate education to be individuals which is their birthright as American citizens.

Really conscientious parents of young deaf children should always make sure that they are maintaining full two-way communication with them. If these parents use the total method to communicate with their children right from infancy, they should begin to see a normal pattern of responses, albeit these may be in gestures or signs as well as oral responses. By "a normal pattern of responses," I mean that the deaf child should parallel a hearing child by first giving incomplete and probably unrecognizable gestures in response, and then gradually progressing to more understandable responses until the child reaches the age of two or three. Then the toddler should be able to express him/herself so that the parents will be able to recognize the child's wants and needs. As long as the child gives reasonable and spontaneous responses, the parents can be sure that they are keeping the channel of communication open both ways, whether manually or orally.

To summarize, deaf children, like all other human beings, need full communication from the time of their birth or loss of hearing in order to develop and grow psychologically and linguistically. This normal development is not possible unless the deaf child is able to participate fully in the give and take of family communication, and to be totally involved in their activities. Since sounds alone are ineffective with hearing impaired children, substitute or supplementary methods must be used for full exchanges of information.

4 The Deaf as a Minority Group

The minority group status of the deaf is producing more numerous and greater problems for them than the handicap itself. This statement becomes more credible when comparing deaf people with other disadvantaged minorities: the blacks, the Chicanos, the American Indians, etc. Deaf people can identify with many of the same problems encountered by these minority groups.

Sue Mitchell in her doctoral dissertation gave an interesting explanation for the present situation of deaf adults:

> The deaf individual has commonly found himself the victim of a self-defeating cycle. In our society, pressures exist to influence minority group members to be the kinds of persons the stereotype say they are. If, on the grounds of perceived inferiority, a segment of the population is provided with a restricted education, poor jobs, and little opportunity for advancement, the conditions have been created for the reinforcement of the belief in inferiority.
>
> The pattern of restrictive attitudes, shown directed toward deaf people in the nineteenth century, had its origin in selective perception and stereotypy to rationalize the actions of the hearing population. The restrictive attitudes in turn created a continuing justification for the economic inequities experienced by the deaf. As an illustration of the self-fulfilling prophecy, such a cycle is an important part of minority-majority relations. Negative expectations are reinforced, providing a basis for further inequities. (p. 130)

McCay Vernon and Bernard Makowsky also delineated the dynamics of the deaf as a minority group fully and forcefully in an article in *The Deaf American* magazine. The majority demands that a minority group conform to its expectations, and at the same time ignores the peculiar problems and needs of that minority group. Thus, in our own case we can say that the great hearing majority is indeed "deaf" to the needs of the deaf!

These problems are compounded by the very nature of deafness. It is so invisible to the casual beholder that the outward behavior of a deaf person resembles that of any ordinary person. It comes as a very great shock when the hearing person discovers a person is deaf. Deafness becomes apparent only when the deaf person begins to converse with someone else on his hands, begins to write on a pad what he wants to say, or indicates that he is deaf when the hearing person attempts to start a conversation with him.

This same shock is what the parents of a deaf child experience when they finally find out what is really wrong. This shock, together with the apparent normalcy of their child, creates a very strong desire on the part of the parents, sometimes approaching an unreasoning obsession, that their deaf child should also act normally—that is, behave like a hearing child. They frequently disregard the deepseated problems and needs of deafness in order to achieve a "pale imitation of a hearing person," at the cost of a happy and fulfilled deaf adult.

Michael Goodman enlarged on this prevailing attitude on the part of the parents of deaf children in a handbook for college instructors as follows:

> The fact that "the deaf child makes his appearance on this mortal scene to all outward appearances as the equal of a hearing child" has caused many deaf children to experience unnecessary suffering and retardation in early life. It is ironic that the problem of adjustment to a child's deafness is often greater in the parents and his family than in the child himself. The people around the deaf child often find it hard to adjust to the situation of having a case of deafness in the family. It makes the parents feel a sense of guilt which they cannot explain. It frustrates them that they cannot communicate with their child. There is a feeling of isolation on both sides, yet an irrational feeling continues to exist that the child can adjust to the hearing world normally in time.
>
> In this way many deaf young children are neglected during the most formative years of their lives. When the deaf child does not

exhibit his deafness, the parents are not embarrassed by him, and the shame or guilt feelings which have afflicted them lie low for the time being. As he follows his parents around, from the super-market to the dry cleaners, he has the outward appearance of any "normal" child. And this is the picture which his parents would like to preserve, whether they know it or not.

The trouble is that this repressive, ignorant, stultifying outlook means that the deaf child might not learn sign language—those ridiculous gestures which draw attention to him as nothing else can—and it means that he might not go to a special school for deaf children soon enough. Let him learn lipreading! Everybody knows that deaf people are good lipreaders! (If it were only true.)

So the situation we have here is that of a child, cut off from com-munication with his family and friends, regarded possibly with shameful feelings by bewildered, ignorant parents who have no no-tion of how to unlock the forces within him, living in a world of complete and unrelieved silence. (pp. 25-26)

After evaluating a selected sample of parents of deaf children, Hilde Schlesinger and Kathryn Meadow had this to say about them in *Deafness and Mental Health: A Developmental Approach:*

These comparisons showed the mothers of deaf children to be significantly more controlling, more intrusive, more didactic, less flexible, and less approving of their children than the mothers of hearing children.

. . . .

The deaf childen's parents verbalized a good deal of frustration and irritation with the impediments to parent-child communica-tion while simultaneously insisting that the deaf child was "really" no different from his hearing sibs. (p. 160)

Many hearing educators cater to this natural preference of the parents for a normally behaving child, and establish educa-tional policies which ignore the real neds of deaf children in order to shape them into molds which are more acceptable to the hearing society. A common practice of those educators is to encourage deaf children to integrate with hearing children in classes and on the playground so as to "normalize" the han-dicapped children. That this philosophy scarcely succeeds is best explained in *Psychological Practices with the Physically Disabled* by James Garrett and Edna Levine:

> The average hearing person has difficulty communicating with the deaf. The hearing person has some normal expectation about how communications should take place, and there is a shock in not being able to communicate naturally. Since this expectancy is not fulfilled, the hearing individual becomes disturbed, irritated, frustrated or embarrassed.
>
> . . . .
>
> What happens when a person finds himself in a disturbing and uncomfortable situation? When we feel unsure and uneasy the natural response often is to try to eliminate the cause of our uneasiness or distress as soon as possible by terminating the event, as in this situation the conversation.
>
> . . . .
>
> As we look at the above situation, we could say for a hearing person, who is distressed or disturbed by the lack of adequate feedback or who withdraws from the situation because the failure to communicate leaves him feeling inadequate, that repeated occurrences would only reinforce this situation and increase the likelihood that when he is again confronted with the opportunity to communicate with a deaf person, he will avoid it.

A deaf acquaintance aptly expressed the deaf person's feelings in such situations: ''A deaf person is more alone among hearing people than he is when being alone.'' What makes this sadder and more infuriating to the deaf adults is that those educators, who have had no better than secondhand experiences with deafness, should be in positions of authority where they have influenced the development of untold thousands of deaf children. They have even resorted to coercion in order to maintain their prestige and philosophy. Mindel and Vernon mentioned this fact in their book on deaf children, *They Grow in Silence:*

> Oralism's adherents will often intimidate or threaten parents to maintain their dominant position. The authors can document instances in which parents were told if they used sign language with their child, they could expect prejudicial treatment by school of-

ficials, to be kept on waiting list excessively long, or to be excluded
from the school system entirely . . . Few parents can stand these
pressures and are eventually brought to their knees. (p. 72)

They, together with their political superiors and parents,
have consistently refused to listen to, let alone consult the only
people who have been through the mill—the deaf themselves.

Fredereick Schreiber, the late Executive Secretary of the National Association of the Deaf, a participant in the *Guest Lecturer
Series,* 1971, at the North Carolina School for the Deaf, said:

. . . it becomes somewhat disheartening to learn that a prominent
educator of the deaf, when asked how her graduates were faring in
the world of work, replied, "That's irrelevant." (p. 53)

Since speech and hearing are the natural modes of communication with people who have normal hearing, they try to
foist them on deaf children. Therefore, the children are compelled to carry on halting communication with a probably
useless remnant of hearing, and whatever segments of speech
are visible to them. They are usually prevented from using any
other means of communication except written English. The rationale has a four-point explanation.

1. *The deaf child will be able to talk like hearing people.* Oral skills
can be divided into two parts: expressive, or speech; and receptive, or speechreading. Therefore, let us examine each aspect
separately.

In order to develop normal speech, the voice has to be continually monitored for volume, pitch, inflection, and pleasant-
ness. Once monitored for a situation, the voice can not be used
in exactly the same way all the time; succeeding and changing
situations require that the voice be readjusted each time, which
can be done only if it is monitored. Without any hearing, or
maybe with some distorted residual hearing, how can a person
monitor his own voice? Thus, even the best deaf talkers have a
peculiar quality of voice, which knowledgeable persons call a
"deafy" voice. An uninitiated hearing person is often startled

to hear this kind of voice, which is a monotone. Without knowing the actual cause, he is most likely to consider it a strange foreign accent.

Unfortunately, in an oral program, not only the child but also the teachers are usually hypnotized into thinking that the deaf child's voice can become natural. Not realizing that her continual contact with deaf children's voices had desensitized and acclimatized her to the unnatural voices, the teacher is easily pleased with progress in the quality of these voices, and in turn is quick to praise and encourage the children.

Thus, these children are encouraged to go out in the world and use their "fine" voices. It is a blow to them when they find that strangers have difficulty understanding them and are sometimes offended by their speech. Although some go on using their speech, others find it too traumatic to attempt to be understood and cease to use their voices in public.

As has been explained in the chapter on communication, speechreading at its best is only educated guesswork. It is a talent which some deaf adults successfully develop into something useful, while others find it a difficult skill to master. It can be compared with breaking an 80 in golf or painting a masterpiece in oils. Speechreading talent has absolutely no correlation with intelligence.

The story given below illustrates the unreliability of speechreading:

> Take the case of a deaf leader, deafened at the age of 10, with excellent speech and lipreading skills which come in very handy for him in his business. He travels extensively; but unpleasant experiences have compelled him to follow a policy which has since then helped him to escape further repetitions of such experiences.
>
> The policy? Each time he buys tickets or asks for reservations over a counter, he writes down his requests on paper and hands it over to the airline representative.

The clerk in turn jots down flight numbers, dates, and times.

Unpleasant experiences? Every time he used his speech to place his request, the airline clerk would automatically answer orally, giving the necessary details which would most of the time contain numbers. The deaf man found that it was very easy to misread lips, and end up with reservations for wrong flights. Then he would have a very difficult time convincing the clerk that he could not hear and that it would be better for the clerk to jot down the needed information so that he could be 100 percent sure before confirming the reservation; the clerk could not understand that one who spoke so well could have a hard time understanding him in turn!

2. *The deaf child will integrate into the hearing community.* As has been stated previously in this chapter, integration with hearing people produces strain and unease due to the fact that communication between deaf people and hearing people is difficult and constrained. Even those hearing persons who are skillful in manual communication find speech to be more relaxing since it is their first method of conversation. I have attended integrated social affairs frequently, and inevitably deaf and hearing persons eventually drift toward their own kind of friends so that toward the end of the evening it is a rare thing to find a group that is still mixed.

In school programs that are integrated, you will usually find deaf children segregated into their own groups on the playground. However, more effective integration occurs when hearing children are given the opportunity to learn manual communication. Then they can talk with deaf students. This is logical, as the hearing youngsters have no obstacle in their way when they learn to communicate with their deaf friends, whereas deaf youngsters would have to surmount an impossibly difficult handicap in order to learn to talk understandably to their hearing friends.

3. *If the deaf child is not taught to be oral, but permitted to use manual* communication, he will likely be isolated in "deaf ghettos."*

This statement is misleading, as the segregation is likely to happen, not because the child is either oral or manual but simply because he is deaf. It is entirely natural for a common handicap to draw people together. Their mutual problems and interests keep them in a body. Thus, not only deaf people, but also blind people, paraplegics, and for that matter, chess players, Catholics, Jehovah's Witnesses, fishermen, golfers, and others find a common bond. It is very likely that, contrary to their teachers' expectations, deaf graduates from programs employing oral methods will seek their own kind for satisfying companionship instead of integrating into the hearing community. For example, the overwhelming majority of graduates of the Clarke School for the Deaf, one of the most widely known institutions still using oralism, marry deaf people.

4. *If deaf children use manual communication, it will interfere with their acquisition of oral skills and good English.*

This rationale, which is of unknown antiquity, has been repeatedly proven invalid by research findings. Meadow, Vernon and Koh, Stuckless and Birch, Montgomery, Stevenson, Quigley and Frisina, Hester, Quigley, Denton, and Moores (in press) found that early manual communication contributed to significantly better academic achievement and often helped improve speechreading abilities. Deaf adults have long known this fact, but it took these recent research discoveries to convince some hearing educators.

Although manual communication has been used by deaf adults in varying guises and degrees, this fact has been consistently ignored by hearing educators who favor the pure oral method of education. These educators have downgraded

*See Glossary, p. 139.

manual communication as being an inferior language, only used by the illiterate deaf, which is far from the truth. Through their efforts and propaganda put out by prestigious organizations, the general public has grown to accept this thesis as being true. It has learned to look down on the deaf who use manual communication, and to give its approbation to those who are able to use some speech and to read lips to some degree. The public tends to equate speech ability with knowledge and intelligence, which is doing the deaf a grave injustice, as nothing can be further from the truth. The attitude and treatment of the deaf as a minority group can be equated with the same treatment by the public of the Chicanos who speak Spanish as their first language, and English as their second.

This brings us to another problem that the deaf have had to contend with—paternalism by hearing educators, which has been a blight upon the educational practices for the deaf for the more than 150 years that we have had formal educational programs in the United States. This attitude has been general among educators working with the deaf, whether they espouse the pure oral philosophy or the more humanitarian one of the combined method.

Paternalism seems to me to be an attitude that is ingrained in hearing persons who have not been intimate with handicapped people long enough to learn to look upon them as people first, and handicapped second. Therefore, when they begin to get acquainted with a group of handicapped people, they are more likely to be conscious of their handicap first, and regard them as a separate class of people. This attitude is strengthened by the communication gap that exists between hearing and deaf people.

The educators supporting the pure oral method seem to be much more blatantly paternalistic than the others, possibly because most of their deaf subjects fail to measure up to their rigid specifications in oral skills, and they are unable to communicate with them manually and get to know them better as

worthwhile individuals. Indeed, one is given to believe that
these teachers have found manual communication too complicated and time consuming to learn, so they have taken the
easier road out by compelling deaf children to come all the
way, over the hurdle of their handicap, to learn their own com-
muniction modes.

The others, who tolerate total communication, are not as of-
fensively paternalistic as the oral method proponents, but they
still regard manual communication as a secondary language
and have been guilty of being paternal in their actions.

These anecdotes which came to me through mutual friends
employed in other schools for the deaf in the nation will serve to
point out what I mean by ''paternalism.''

> In at least two schools in the Midwest the principals
> employ a double standard for conduct. Whenever hear-
> ing parents come to visit and inquire about their deaf
> children in the programs, these principals would use
> their best brand of behavior: courteous and helpful.
> But, when deaf parents of deaf children in the same pro-
> grams come for exactly the same purpose, these prin-
> cipals would be short and brusque with them; they
> would not hesitate to ''tell them off,'' thus making them
> feel that they had no right in coming and questioning
> the school's actions with their children.
>
> In an Eastern school, which is inclined toward
> oralism although ostensibly practicing the ''combined
> method,'' there is a speech therapist who seems to have
> no use for deaf adults. At least, she has never bothered
> to learn manual communication. She seems to regard
> manual conversations as being beneath her notice, for
> she has been irritating the deaf staff members by break-
> ing into manual conversations that they hold with hear-
> ing staff members without so much as saying, ''by your
> leave,'' to start her own conversations with the hearing
> colleagues. Being drawn and quartered would be too

good for that therapist, for by her actions she unconsciously implies that deaf people are beneath her notice. Yet, she does not hesitate to make her living from deaf children!

Paternalism can be unconscious, as this story will illustrate:

It involves a couple of hearing staff members at my school who have never shown any attitude toward me other than mutual courtesy and respect. However, at a school event I was engaged in a conversation with a well-known hearing educator who was visiting the school. He is the son of deaf parents and treats deaf people as his equals. Just then the above-mentioned hearing colleagues came up with another hearing visitor and broke into our conversation. Subtly elbowing me aside, they started an animated conversation with my hearing friend so that I was left on the outside to gaze upon them. It was not until that conversation languished that they thought of permitting the second visitor to greet me. You can imagine my unalloyed delight when the first-mentioned hearing guest suddenly took off to greet a dear deaf friend of his who happened to come into the room just then. It really did my ego good to see the group of startled hearing persons watch the hearing visitor clamp the deaf friend in a bear hug!

Paradoxically, those hearing educators who regard deaf people with a superior air seem to command greater awe and respect from deaf children, for there is a subtle communicative barrier between them, which the hearing teachers do not bother to remove. Like colonials in white suits, they gain "respect" from the natives through a distancing, ritualistic one-upmanship.

Unfortunately few of these educators have intimately mingled with, or made the slightest effort to know the "grass-roots" deaf adults; they are usually ignorant of what is going on in the adult deaf world. In all the years I have spent in the deaf community, which means most of my life, I have noted the presence of hearing educators in the local club of the deaf probably less than five times. However, they do occasionally attend the more salubrious church, charity, and state association affairs. And, the hearing educators at my school have been considered to be among the most progressive and democratic teachers in the country! Using this as a standard of comparison, it is obvious that most educators do not even bother to make their presence noticed in the local adult deaf communities.

These educators would never consider consulting deaf adults, nor think of appointing them to policy-making positions. Nor would they willingly create situations where hearing parents of deaf children can get into contact with, and get acquainted with deaf adults so that they can learn what sort of adults their deaf children will grow up to be. They never look upon the deaf as anything other than second-class citizens.

Even though the system of educating deaf children in the United States is full of faults and personnel who impede optimum achievement by deaf children, deaf adults in our country enjoy, by comparison, the best standard of living in the world. Therefore, it seems the height of irony that the Alexander Graham Bell Association should sponsor a Foreign Lecturer Series in which foreign authorities in the field are invited to tour the United States with all their expenses paid to tell about educational practices overseas which have been instrumental in keeping their deaf people in virtual peonage. One man in particular, Dr. Anthony van Uden, from the Netherlands, stated in a press interview that sign language is only used by imbeciles!

However, thanks to the militancy of the blacks, the Chicanos, the American Indians, and other minority groups, the large majority who hear have begun to be aware of the rights of deaf people as a minority group, and to realize that they have a vital message which has long been ignored by the hearing.

Director of Public Information for the NAD, Edward C. Carney, formerly Executive Director of the Council of Organizations Serving the Deaf (which is no longer an active organization), made this statement before the Subcommittee on the Handicapped of the Senate Committee on Labor and Public Welfare relative to Vocational Rehabilitation Amendments of 1972 on June 6, 1972:

> The provision for consumer representation is especially meaningful. Already, within the Department of Health, Education, and Welfare, it has been shown that the most effective programs are those which have included in the planning stages persons for whose benefits the programs were designed. Deaf people, as well as other minority groups, have needs and desires which are not understood readily by persons who have not themselves experienced the particular handicap or disadvantage. Involvement of the consumer generally has resulted in more realistic planning and meaningful implementation of programs of assistance. This should be evidenced even more convincingly when deaf persons are afforded the opportunity for input at the time of program planning. At least one prominent author has referred to the deaf as the ''most misunderstood of the sons of men.'' With direct involvement of the deaf consumer, as would be provided under this bill, the door to understanding would be opened; it is reasonable to expect that understanding would be achieved both ways. That is, the deaf person not only would be better understood, but would, himself, better understand the many beneficial services available to him. (pp. 1061-1062)

It was, therefore, not because of total communication, advanced technology, nor improved hearing aids, but because the deaf consumer has been increasingly involved in governmental planning of the various programs for their benefit, that American deaf citizens have been securing additional rights. They, however, have a long road to travel before they can achieve first class citizenship.

Perhaps the one who is the most responsible for these enlightened changes is Dr. Boyce R. Williams, director of Deafness and Communicative Disorders Office in the Rehabilitation Services Administration. He was the first deaf person to achieve a high-level position in the Federal government where he could make policy changes which got the ball rolling for needed services to the deaf as well as to secure more effective participation by the deaf. It was thus that the National Association of the Deaf grew immensely in political power and influence, assisted by Federal grants, many of which originated in Dr. Williams' office.

Now we have, or have had, deaf directors of the Office of Deafness and Communicative Disorders, R.S.A., American Deafness and Rehabilitation Association, American Coalition of Citizens with Disabilities, Inc., Convention of American Instructors of the Deaf, Council on Education of the Deaf, the Registry of Interpreters for the Deaf, the Communicative Skills Program, and the Media Services and Captioned Films office. Gallaudet College, California State University at Northridge, University of Arizona, and many schools for the deaf have appointed qualified deaf persons to positions of authority and influence.

Although the picture is brightening for the deaf as minority group citizens, we still have many hearing people who are fighting this trend. Some of them may be sincere in their beliefs, but the others are probably struggling to maintain the *status quo* so that they may keep their own prestige and influence, not to mention sources of their bread and butter. The Alexander Graham Bell Association is notable in this respect. In their fight to maintain their strict oral philosophy they have formed the Oral Deaf Adults Section, whose members are proudly reciting their own successes in various careers without resorting to the use of manual communication. Although they are not educators and have not had contact with deaf youngsters with various educational problems, they do not hesitate to advise on educational matters. Unfortunately, they have sold out many future deaf adults by singing their siren song to gullible parents, who then desperately try to mold their own deaf children after these successful oral adults. The many resulting failures do not justify the few successes. It would be well if those parents would stop and ponder that while the Oral Deaf Adults Section has about 250 members, at the best estimate, the National Association of the Deaf lists about 18,000 deaf adults, many of whom were oral failures, who are now happy and productive members of the deaf comunity, as well as society at large.

5 Traditional Educational Methods

Before a person can begin to comprehend what sort of a person the average deaf adult in our society is, he should first know what traditonal means have been used to educate him. Perhaps a little history is now in order.

One of the most definitive works on deafness is Harry Best's book, *Deafness and the Deaf in the United States.* He mentioned two educators in Europe who were the most influential in the development of educational methods used with the deaf. First was Samuel Heinicke, who started the first public school for the deaf in Leipsig, Germany, in 1778. He was responsible for bringing the oral method into favor, and may be said to be the "father of oralism." Another was Charles Michel Abbé de l'Épée, who founded the first regular school in Europe in 1755. He was influential in introducing sign language as a method of teaching the deaf, although he used the oral method first with young deaf children. He was probably responsible for the methods first used in America, since our benefactor, Thomas Hopkins Gallaudet, went to Paris and learned teaching methods from Abbé de l'Épée's successor, Abbé Roch-Ambroise Cucurron Sicard.

The first permanent school established in the United States was the one founded by Thomas Gallaudet in Hartford, Connecticut. He became involved with a little deaf daughter of a physician, Alice Cogswell, whose friends decided to organize in order to start a school for deaf children. They sent Mr. Gallaudet to Europe to learn the methods of teaching the deaf. He went first to a private school in London run by the family of Thomas Braidwood, but found that they intended to keep their methods a secret. So, he went to Paris where Abbé Sicard gladly demonstrated the methods used at his school, which included manual communication. Mr. Gallaudet observed closely, and brought with him to America a young deaf teacher, Laurent Clerc.

It is noteworthy that from the very beginning of formal education for the deaf in the United States the concept of having deaf teachers of deaf children has met with acceptance, whereas in other parts of the world such teachers are rare. It also should be mentioned that many of our schools for the deaf were founded by deaf men: Florida (Thomas H. Coleman); Gallaudet Day School (Delos A. Simpson); New Mexico (Lars M. Larson); Kansas (Philip A. Emery); Oregon (William S. Smith); North Dakota (A. R. Spear); Arizona (H. C. White); and Virginia, Newport News (W. C. Ritter). It would be interesting research to ascertain just how the control of these schools was taken or shifted away from these deaf gentlemen and given to hearing educators who either worked for, or permitted, oralism to gain ascendancy over manual communication.

Thus, the "combined method,"* using both oral and manual methods, came first to the United States, and this method found favor in most of the state public schools which were subsequently founded.

However, as the instruction of the deaf grew and developed in America, hearing educators began to oppose the use of sign language, and to believe in the greater efficacy of the oral method. This belief was strengthened by the fact that this method was more widely used in Europe. Therefore, in 1843, Horace Mann and Samuel Gridley Howe of Massachusetts visited Germany where they observed the methods used by Samuel Heinicke. They came back favoring the oral means of teaching the deaf. This naturally found more and more favor among hearing educators and parents who found manual communication to be strange and disturbing to them.

---

*See Dr. Sue Mitchell's comments on the combined method on following pages.

Therefore, a little after the middle of the nineteenth century, agitation for the pure oral method became more pronounced, and the first of the well-known oral schools was established. This is the Clarke School for the Deaf, now at Northampton, Massachusetts. At about the same time, the forerunner of the present Lexington School was founded in New York City. In 1869, the first day school for the deaf, the Horace Mann School, was started in Boston. This started the oral trend for day school programs for the deaf all over the country.

The oral movement in the education of the deaf in the United States went forward with rapidity and vigor, and special organizations were started to encourage and foster oral endeavors and to frown upon the use of signs and fingerspelling. The largest organization was the American Association for the Promotion of the Teaching of Speech to the Deaf, which later became the Alexander Graham Bell Association of the Deaf. Its Volta Bureau in Washington, D.C., has been very influential in promoting the pure oral methods of instructing the deaf.

Dr. Sue Mitchell has perhaps explained the methods of teaching during the years before total communication was introduced as well as any one else could.

Essentially, the key to the 1867-1952 period was the philosophical dichotomy between educators adhering to the oral method exclusively and those using the combined method. Those of the pure oralist tradition believed that the deaf child who was extensively exposed to speech exclusively would, if he were of at least average intelligence, learn adequate oral communication and be successfully returned to the hearing world. The combined method theoretically employed the communication method or methods which were best suited to the development of an individual child. Since the combined method varied so much from one place to another, the best general explanation would be that within a school employing this method, more than just instruction by oral means was given. One school perhaps used speech accompanied by fingerspelling, while another had rigidly separated oral and

manual programs functioning side by side. In a school of the latter
type, children were placed in a unit being taught via the sign
language only if they appeared unable to succeed orally. (p. 52)

The reader should understand that all these initial efforts in
educating the deaf and the methods used were determined by
people who by virtue of their hearing had only vicarious experience with deafness. That the deaf were not consulted
should also be understood and appreciated; they were, for the
most part, uneducated recipients of compassion and charity.

Unfortunately, up to very recently, these traditional
methods (combined and oral) were general in the United States
schools for the deaf. Also during the same period, no deaf persons were hired as teachers in some schools, and in many of the
other schools, deaf teachers were compelled to accept lower pay
scales than hearing teachers even though their extra-curricular
duties might be much heavier. No deaf persons, with a few
notable exceptions, such as Arthur L. Roberts, J. Schuyler
Long, Tom L. Anderson, Tom Dillon, and James N. Orman,
were permitted to possess and enjoy positions where they could
participate in decision and policy making.

As recently as 1954, a subcommittee conducting a study to
determine competencies needed by teachers of the deaf, under
the direction of Dr. Romaine Mackie, Specialist, the United
States Office of Education, Department of Health, Education,
and Welfare, submitted a report to the Conference of the Executives of American Schools for the Deaf. In that report included in the *Minutes of the 26th Regular Meeting* was a section
which was disputed by some members of the committee. It
follows:

> We turn now to an unresolved difference of opinion in our com-
> mittee concerning the requirement that the teacher of the deaf
> must speak and hear normally (and obviously is free from any
> disfigurement or bodily movement which could interfere with
> lipreading). Those of us whose names are listed immediately below

this section support unreservedly the requirement of normal
speech and hearing because we believe that they are necessary for
the acquisition and application of the knowledge and abilities
recommended in this report.

> Marguerite Stoner
> Alice Streng
> Serena Davis
> Clarence D. O'Connor
> S. Richard Silverman

Three members of the Competencies Committee did not
sign that section. They were Thomas H. Poulos, Hugo
Schunhoff, and Richard G. Brill. Byron B. Burnes, who was
then the President of the National Association of the Deaf, obtained permission from Dr. Howard Quigley, the president of
the Conference, to address the group on this section. The
ultimate result was a resolution rejecting outright the above
segment of the report, and it was passed by the Conference.
Fortunately for the American deaf, we had enough hearing
friends in the Conference to defeat an abominable effort by
members of the hearing majority to keep the deaf minority
from taking part in determining their own destiny, for the Conference did not have any members who were deaf themselves.
An interesting footnote to this was the fact that the president of
the National Association of the Deaf was not even listed among
the guests of the Conference in the minutes.

Almost all teacher training programs during the same period
followed the pure oral philosophy, and refused to permit the
trainees to learn manual communication even though 95 percent of the deaf adults use it all the time.

Even in the schools following the "combined method"
philosophy, the methods of instruction in the lower grades were
purely oral. The deaf pupils were only allowed to change to
"manual classes" when they were proven to be failures in the
oral method, usually during their adolescence. These older
pupils were generally considered to be brain damaged, aphasic,

or "slow," by their teachers. Thus, many bright and capable youngsters were labeled failures—and after living in a climate of failures, they inevitably became failures in everything else. Thus, incalculable damage was done not only to their self-image but also to their capabilities for optimum achievement toward desirable careers.

It is infuriating and painful for any compassionate human being to see impatient parents and teachers struggle with recalcitrant deaf children, trying to make them utter recognizable sounds. The most reprehensible thing about foisting a pure oral philosophy of communication upon a deaf child is its repressive character. It is extremely distressing to observe a hefty adult clamping a little deaf child's jaws so that he can not look in any direction other than directly at the perspiring grown-up in order for him either to demonstrate to the child how a word should be spoken or to compel the little being to read his lips and get what he was trying to tell the child. This practice has given some deaf youngsters such a psychological tic that they find it impossible to look directly into anyone's eyes.

It is a wonder, indeed, that there is not more psychological destruction than there is. I am quite sure that if I had not had deaf parents, I would have become emotionally disturbed. Any smart, self-respecting individual would not have accepted such indignities without protesting. It is a sad thing that many deaf children are in such a helpless position that when they protest they are immediately cracked down on by offended educators for exhibiting anti-social behavior.

Here are several cases of maladjustment which are examples of what has occurred when children were restricted to one method of communication, and as a consequence, deprived of meaningful communication.

Ralph and James were deaf children of "self-made" fathers. They were confined to programs using the oral method until they became too old for the educators and fathers to conceal the fact that they were "oral failures." Then they were admitted to a state residential school. By that time the damage had been done, and only instruction of a terminal type could be offered to them so that they would find it of some value when they left school. Since then both fathers have been trying to transfer their guilt to the school, blaming the school for their sons' shortcomings.

Charles was the son of a well-to-do farmer, who apparently could not accept his only male offspring's deafness. He made no attempt to establish communication with Charles, who happened to have very little talent for speech and lipreading. Although Charles was handsome, athletic, and smart, he refused to conform to the residential school's rules and policies, with the result that he was continually in hot water. I feel that it was his way of rebelling against his father's repressive silence.

Dennis was the eldest of four sons, and the only deaf child of a domineering mother. In her drive toward normalcy for Dennis, his mother placed him in an oral program at first. Finding that there was no satisfactory secondary program for him other than what a residential school was offering, she begrudgingly permitted him to be exposed to manual communication. Being quite intelligent, Dennis made good progress and graduated with a good record. However, this has not stopped his mother's continuing diatribes against the residential school and manual communication. Dennis' personality is showing a definite effect from his mother's hectoring; he is withdrawn and hesitant in his actions, and stutters even in manual communication.

Although Randall grew to be a big and heavy-set boy, he continued to be closely watched and protected by his mother. She refused to leave him to the tender mercies of the dormitories at a residential school. She bused him about 15 miles each way every day. She came to the school well before the dismissal time so that she could whisk him away before he could go as far as the dormitory grounds. Subsequently, he developed a very passive personality, and when he graduated, he quickly disappeared from sight.

Both Ted and Jerry came to a residential school from the same oral day class program. Ted was transferred from the day class program out of despair on the part of his parents, for Ted was an oral failure. He could not learn anything at all, and when he reached the residential school, he was literally dumb because he could not communicate in any way at all. Jerry was quite the opposite, for he developed the best oral skills of all the children at the day class program, and his teachers touted his skills, taking him on demonstration trips, etc.

However, Ted found himself when he discovered manual communication, and soon was making astonishing progress. He caught up with his age level, and displayed an extraordinary bent for mathematics. His language developed at such a rate that he was writing fairly adequate English at the time of his graduation from the school. He also went on to attend Gallaudet College, where his mathematical talent was recognized, and was given special attention. He is now holding a lucrative job as a programmer for the IBM Corporation.

On the other hand, Jerry was found to be educationally retarded and place in a class for slow learners, where he made satisfactory progress. He was definitely not collegiate material.

This is meant to be critical of the oral method, and of the oral teachers' attitude toward these two boys. Ted almost lost out entirely because they did not see anything in him.

In defense of a single method of communication, one may go to *The Volta Review* magazine, and find these rationalizations:

George W. Fellendorf, of the Alexander Graham Bell (A.G.B.) Association:

> The father and mother who recognize that the easy way is not the oral way and still dedicate themselves to this philosophy are probably inviting a certain amount of additional frustration, concern, and worry into their home as a part of the price. . . . There is effort involved in the oral approach, and the price may be high in meeting the demands it places upon the family and the child. (p. 352)

Chris R. Hoerr, III, also of the A.G.B. Association:

> Patience is a key objective and trait that must be developed by all parents of deaf children. . . . Slow academic progress in a child's early years often leads us to believe that he is a "slow learner." Our impatience might suggest changing the approach or method of his instruction. . . . Many parents have not developed the extra patience that the teaching of speech and lipreading demands. They have changed to the "easy way out" method of education (sometimes referred to as T.C.) and have enrolled in a fingerspelling and sign language class themselves so that they can communicate "more easily" with their own child. . . . Patience is the key ingredient in turning the NOW generation into the THEN generation as far as the education of deaf children is concerned. (pp. 332-333)

Patience, indeed! If you would go out in the streets with me, you would see too many deaf adults who have been wrecked by too much patience and oralism during their young, sensitive years. The price is too high to pay!

The proponents of oralism naturally place very heavy emphasis upon the training of young deaf children in speech and lipreading. However, their philosophy of teaching these skills without using the additional help of other aspects of total communication* has been self-defeating because these children

*See Chapter 6.

usually have no background of experience, whether visual or auditory, upon which they might be able to build additional proficiencies in oral skills.

Now, with the introduction and acceptance of the total communication concept, the teachers are finding it more effective, more relaxing, and less traumatic to teach deaf youngsters oral skills after they are given the opportunity to acquire the necessary knowledge and background by total communication. The children are then growing aware of the need to acquire oral skills, and at the same time have the necessary vocabulary and language to connect up with sounds being taught. Armed with this knowledge, they are able to recognize more words on the lips. Speech therapists are also finding it easier and more fruitful to use manual communication in correcting speech and drilling in speechreading. Although this may be surprising to some, it is not so to the deaf and other knowledgeable persons that deaf children are developing even better speech and lipreading this way than they have under the older and more repressive oral philosophy.

Schlesinger and Meadow mentioned this fact in their book entitled *Deafness and Mental Health*:

> . . . it seemed of extreme practical significance that younger day school children who had some facility with manual communication scored at a much higher level on the Lipreading Inventory than did any of the other groups. (p. 129)

In addition to contributing to better lipreading, early manual communication, in adjunct with other methods, also encourages optimum development of personalities. This may be proved by picking out girls and boys with outgoing temperments and leadership qualities from the student body at any school, which either practices or permits total communication. A higher percent of these students generally prove to have either deaf parents or hearing parents who have established total communication with them very early.

On the other hand, the hearing authorities of traditional educational programs always made it a point to assure the parents of their deaf students that the school "does not teach them the sign language," which was unfortunately true.

The deaf pupils at the schools using the "combined method" pick up their sign language haphazardly outside the classroom, hence starting with a bastard mixture of conventional, homemade, and slang signs. Eventually, as they grew up and achieved their own spheres of friends, they developed systems of signs which were used for the remainder of their lives. Thus, the more educated youngsters would use more formal signs and a greater amount of fingerspelling while the less educated students would be content with a more elementary form of the sign language, using fingerspelling less.

The above facts bring forth another vital fact concerning traditional educational practices used with the deaf up to the last few years, one which should be underlined and constantly reiterated: In all educational programs the deaf child had been exposed to no other than oral methods during his early and formative years. As any average deaf person knows, oral communication is elliptic, halting, impeditive, and frustrating. This restrictive communication used with very young and untutored deaf children is contrary to the psychological precept that the best time to educate children is during their first few years of life.

In *Hearings before the Subcommittee on the Handicapped* Mr. Edward C. Carney had this to say about the rejection of oralism by young deaf children:

> . . . important factors (for deaf persons being "low achieving")
> would necessarily include: . . . rejection, on the part of the child, of
> an educational system based solely upon an oral approach. Oral
> communication, to the exclusion of any alternative system, can be
> a frustrating and exceedingly difficult experience, particularly to
> an emotionally high-strung child. In the absence of any language
> skills which permit him to comprehend an explanation of the

ultimate advantages of acquiring oral communication skills, and faced with the determination of young and insecure teachers who feel under pressure to conform rigidly to the established system lest they (the teachers) be judged by the authorities to be unqualified to produce positive results, the child rebels. This rebellion may be manifested in any number of ways, and most frequently in varying degrees of emotional disturbance. To some of them, their only defense or possible course of retaliatory action is to slow down or completely suspend conscious learning. They frequently cannot articulate their own motives, but in their innocence the results are personally satisfactory on an immediate basis. Only later, or perhaps never, do they realize the long-range adverse consequences to themselves. (p. 1151)

The blame for the inadequate education that the deaf have been getting has been laid at the door of manual communication for far too long. It is about time that we shift the blame and lay it at the right door: the lack of sufficient communication flowing freely and easily between the teacher and student!

That these restrictive educational methods have continued for so long is due to the existence of a vicious circle of circumstances. The education of the deaf was started by hearing people because, of course, there were no educated deaf people in the first place. We owe it all to those philanthropic people that we are getting any education at all. However, instead of developing the educational methods for greater effectiveness toward the goal of developing happy, well-adjusted and productive deaf citizens, the hearing persons who have been in the saddle of authority have placed the greatest emphasis upon molding deaf children into acceptable facsimiles of hearing people, i.e., themselves. This travesty of an education has produced thousands and thousands of inadequate deaf adults who have been unable to make themselves heard in order to air their grievances. They have not been taught sufficiently well to be able to express themselves plainly and vigorously in clear and understandable English, let alone in intelligible speech. Nor were they taught to read and understand.

Mitchell stated in her doctoral dissertation:

> Centuries of viewing the deaf as idiots and to be avoided had left a legacy of distance and distaste. Approaches calculated to appeal to religious fervor or generous impulses emphasized the difference between the deaf and the hearing, not the the similarities.
>
> Because there was such a small body of general knowledge about the deaf, statements by educators of the deaf were authoritarian. Their control was unusually absolute because community interest and direction was uniquely absent. The relationship between the hearing educators of the deaf and all deaf children and adults was a paternalistic one. In keeping with the missionary frame of reference, the hearing educators were paternalistic because they generally believed the possession of hearing provided a superiority of intellect, judgment, and background. (p. 34)

To carry the above thesis further, let me quote the following from *Hearing and Deafness* pertaining to the desirability of speech and speechreading by two hearing authorities, Hallowell Davis and S. Richard Silverman:

> For some educators, speech is a subject to be taught like a foreign language to those who can "benefit" from it. Practice and atmosphere are not aimed at vitalizing speech for the child. Rather, speech is viewed as an eminently desirable but not essential skill to cultivate. For others (including ourselves), a corollary to the proposition of universality of opportunity to learn speech is inescapable: speech is a basic means of communication and hence is a vital mechanism of adjustment to the communicating world around us. Therefore, we set the stage for the child everywhere—in the home, on the playground, in the schoolroom—from the moment we learn that he is deaf, so that speech eventually becomes meaningful, significant, and purposeful for him at all times . . . Only constant practice and actual use of speech will develop fully the deaf child's latent ability to communicate by speech.
>
> . . . .
>
> The inadequacy of our formal tools for assessment of the ability to speechread need not deter us from suggesting the following guides to practice in developing this valuable skill in deaf children:
>
> 1. An atmosphere of oral communication must be created and maintained.

2. Even if the child is not expected to understand every word of a spoken message, he should be talked to and he should be encouraged to take advantage of situational clues.

3. Speechreading should be reinforced by other sensory clues whenever practical. (pp. 429, 442)

Thus, hearing authorities who have had only vicarious acquaintance with deafness, who do not know sign language, and who know little about living with deafness are deciding what is the best for deaf children. Only the advice given in the last sentance above takes into consideration the fact that the child can not hear so that he can monitor his own speech and listen to the others' speech. The other statements gloss over this inescapable fact! And, so deaf children struggle on, perhaps perplexed that they can not communicate in any easier way.

In *Language and Education of the Deaf* Herbert Kohl questions the reliability of lipreading:

This lipreading is the only direct way a profoundly deaf child can have access to the linguistic world of the hearing. Yet by itself lipreading is hardly adequate for learning English from or perceiving it upon the lips of others. Such dissimilar pairs of words as "cart" and "yarn" and "green" and "red" are practically identical in visual appearance. Nor can a word which is formed from sounds at the back of the mouth—"hit" is an example—be lipread. Neither children nor adults can learn the patternings of sounds that are necessary for an understanding of even the most basic phonemic contrasts in English from lipreading alone. Hester suggests that "Language facility may be one of the most important keys to success in lipreading." Further there is no correlation between intelligence and lipreading ability or, more important, between achievement and lipreading ability. (p. 10)

And, yet, in some educational programs there still exists an authoritarian, paternalistic attitude by hearing educators toward deaf children, not to mention toward deaf adults! In such an atmosphere, deaf children frequently suffer from having new teachers who have not yet developed empathy for deafness, older teachers who are frozen into oral-traditional methods of instruction, or incompetent teachers who have failed in public schools and escaped into the little known world of the education of the deaf.

A good example of such children would be a boy who was admitted to one of the programs in Southern California which follow the total communication philosophy. He had come from a program in the Southeast which had his I.Q. put down as 65. His mentality and behavior were such that the new place decided to re-test his intelligence. This time he scored 120.

Jean was another example of the authoritarian philosophy of oralism. She attended an oral day school in an industrial city. Although her residual hearing was better than average, and she achieved a fairly good speech and developed usuable lipreading skills with the aid of her hearing, her academic achievement was not outstanding. When she left school, she led a lonely life since there were not too many schoolmates who were good company for her. Then, she discovered "manual" deaf adults and manual communication. Her life opened up and she led a happy and active social life. Then she met and married a man who could not speak or read lips even to save his own life.

Although happy now, Jean still regrets that she did not have early manual communication which might have enhanced her academic progress. One day she ran into a former teacher, who had risen to being a director of a teacher training program in a nearby university. At a luncheon she wondered out loud to the teacher as to why she did not have Genevieve, an old school chum who was an oral failure, transferred to the state residential school where Genevieve could have made better academic progress under a more liberal philosophy. "Let's not talk about her," was the teacher's only reply.

Here is an example of the misconceptions which are widely
held by teachers trained in oralism.

There was a state-wide workshop for teachers of the
deaf at the University of California in Santa Barbara
one summer. There my wife Dorothy and I ran into two
charming young ladies who taught day classes in small
towns. Since Dorothy possessed all the oral skills in the
family, she intercepted the conversational ball and kept
it passing back and forth. However, the inevitable im-
passe occurred: my wife failed to make the ladies
understand what she was saying, so she turned to me
and asked me to write down what she was trying to say.
I complied, and handed the pad to one of the ladies.
You can imagine my surprise and discomfort when she
exclaimed, ''You have perfect language. I don't have to
correct a single thing!''

Naturally, I was somewhat nettled at this, so I went
on to impress these young ladies with my command of
English and to try a little dry humor on them. I was in
for another surprise.

The same young lady said in a wondering tone to her
friend, ''Why, he has a sense of humor!'' This compelled me to go on and say still more drily that I needed a
sense of humor to be able to live with my wife. The lady
really laughed out loud, but I could swear that there
was a tinge of wonderment in her laugh.

At the same workshop, a conscientious and troubled
young man called a rump session of teachers on the high
school level. It seemed that his big problem was inadequate materials for his deaf youngsters. He said that his
students were not benefited by what he had, and asked
us to help him pool better materials for mutual use by
other oral teachers of high school age children. I do not
know what stopped me from jumping up and shouting,

"You fools! What's the use of searching for better materials if you can't communicate the concepts to the kids!"

Vernon, in an article in *The Illinois Advance,* reported on the failure of the prevailing education practices used with deaf children as follows:

> The results of the education of the deaf are disgraceful, as the following information will show:
>
> I. *Boatner and McClure Study.* In 1965 a study was done which included 93 percent of all pupils enrolled in schools for the deaf in the United States who were 16 years old or older and who were leaving school. Thirty percent of these youths were functionally illiterate. Only five percent achieved a tenth grade or better level. Of these youth, 60 percent were at grade level 5.3 or below.
>
> II. *Wrightstone, Aronow and Muskowitz Study.* In 1959 they studied 73 school programs involving 53 percent of all deaf school-age children. They found that from the age of 10 years of 16 years, the average gain in reading was less than one year. Furthermore, the average reading score for a 16-year-old deaf youth was grade level 3.4.
>
> III. *Schein and Bushnaq Study.* They found that admissions into college of deaf youth were only one-tenth the percent of admissions into college of normally hearing students. For example, if 40 percent of the normally hearing get into college, then only four percent of the deaf get into college.

It is also unfortunate that inadequate education has created as well the paradoxical state of complacence among the short-changed deaf adults. To put it simply, a great many under-educated deaf adults have never had the chance to delve deeply beneath the surface veneer of everyday competence and to discover the unmined riches of in-depth knowledge and culture. Therefore, they do not know nor care about what they are missing by following a life where they are able to earn a living just adequate for them to exist and enjoy a few superficial amusements or hobbies. Theater, Shakespeare, foreign cultures, *The Atlantic Monthly,* and such areas of appreciation are not for them. And so, they do not even know in what ways their education has failed them!

6 Total Communication

Rationale for Total Communication

Total communication, or "the total approach," has been called many things, from highly complimentary comments to epithets of downright insult. The most frequently quoted definition is that of Margaret Kent, former principal of the Maryland School for the Deaf, which was used by Ottinger in an article in *The Deaf American:*

> . . . the right of a deaf child to use all forms of communication to develop language competence. This includes the full spectrum of child devised gestures, speech, formal signs, fingerspelling, speechreading, reading, and writing. To every deaf child should also be provided the opportunity to learn to use any remnant of residual hearing he may have by employing the best possible electronic equipment for amplifying sound. (pp. 3-6)

Many people have called total communication "a method," along with oral, combined, Rochester, and other methods. In an editorial in *The California News* I gave my viewpoint as follows:

> I conceive of total communication not so much as a method as it is a philosophy—a way of thinking which is rational, kind, considerate, and sensitive to the needs of deaf children. In my way of thinking, total communication is any method or a combination of two or more methods of conveying a desired message to a hearing impaired person such that he is able to understand 100 percent of the message. And, he should also be able to express himself so that his *vis-a-vis* will understand him 100 percent. In the latter case, since the person in question is the one who is handicapped, adjustments should be made by the *vis-a-vis* so that he is able to receive communication 100 percent from the handicapped person. (p. 8)

I would like to go one step further in defining total communication: When the doctrine of total communication is followed, every restraint is removed from the communicative media that are used by deaf children; they are not only allowed to use communicative methods with which they are the most comfortable, but others use the same means to communicate with them, thus establishing a comfortable and meaningful relationship with the handicapped children. No longer are deaf children a group of human beings who have been compelled to limit their communication to a method that is extremely artificial and restraining them; with the total communication concept they are now permitted to gain that optimum education which is their birthright.

For far too long fumbling hearing persons have dictated terms to children about whose handicap they either have a faint conception or hold very misleading theories. Dr. Mervin Garretson, the Special Assistant to the President for Advocacy, Gallaudet College, Washington, D.C., related the following anecdote in a talk on total communication which he presented in California.

> An elderly man in a large eastern metropolis became seriously ill and was rushed to a hospital where the diagnosis was quite bleak. It was felt that the old guy should be with relatives or close friends during what well might be his final days of life. It developed that he had no known living relatives and could give only one name—that of a boyhood friend, but he did not know his present whereabouts. The hospital staff decided to initiate a search for this unknown gentleman, practically combing the entire country. In time the man was located, flown to the city, and rushed to the hospital where he discovered his old friend under the oxygen tent. The sick man tried to talk but words would not come. He waved feebly for a pencil and paper which were quickly given to him. Writing laboriously, he passed away with the paper still clutched in his hand. After the doctor had pronounced him dead, they pried the paper from his hand. He had scrawled: ''Please get your foot off my oxygen hose.''

Thus, well-meaning but misinformed hearing authorities have held their collective foot on deaf children's communicative ''hose,'' and figuratively killed their chances for an optimum education and a subsequently rich and rewarding life as self-sufficient and well adjusted deaf adults. Whether a deaf child has the opportunity for total communication or follows a traditional means of education, he will most likely develop into an adult who may have very little use, if any at all, for the smattering of oral skills which might have been so laboriously drilled into him during most of his school years, and which have occupied most of the traditional educators' time and effort, as well as countless volumes of printed matter and the expenditure of millions of public dollars.

It would be interesting to contemplate as to how much the products of educational programs stressing oralism are making use of their own skills. The epitome of success in making oral communication the way of life seems to be membership in the Oral Deaf Adults Section of the Alexander Graham Bell Association. The Section, however, boasts of only about 250 members at the best estimate. Even if we consider this number or even double this number as being the number of those successful oral adults who do not bother to join the O.D.A.S., there are still many thousands more yet to be reckoned for. As an active member of the deaf community, I have made the acquaintance of thousands who came from pure oral programs to join the society of the deaf who use total communication, and I have run across or heard about many more who have become recluses because they have failed to find happiness and satisfaction in the hearing society with their limited oral skills, and either through pressure from their families or their own hangups, can not use manual communication. So, how can one justify the vast amount of time and money devoted to the single-minded pursuit of oral excellence?

On the other hand, the use of total communication, or rather, free expression with the manual communication sector of total communication, by younger deaf children has resulted in the normal or near normal development of these children not only in language skills but also in other competencies. There have been several studies which prove the value of early manual communication.

Although the use of total communication in preschool and early school years is comparatively recent, the great difference in the achievement rate of the deaf children has been quickly noted, to the great satisfaction of their educators and parents.

On my field trips to observe total communication in action with younger deaf children at the Maryland School for the Deaf in Frederick, at the Madison School* in Santa Ana, California, and at the Arroyo School in Simi Valley, California, I saw nothing but enthusiastic praise of the philosophy by the teachers, many of whom had struggled with the traditional oral philosophy before.

The latest evaluative reports of three programs following total communication philosophy with little deaf children continue to substantiate the earlier reports on manual communication among younger deaf children—that these deaf children achieve at a normal or even better than normal rate. I believe that it would interest hearing parents even more to know that these deaf children have not suffered any loss of their oral skills, and in some cases have done even better.

My Total Communication Philosophy

I do not claim to be an authority on the education of deaf children. I have been deaf all my life and I have taught for most of my adult life; therefore, I have some thoughts on what should be done to provide maximum eductional opportunities for deaf youngsters.

For years I have realized that communication must be broadened and made easier during the earlier years so that deaf children could cope with their communicative needs in order to learn, but I have despaired that hearing educators would ever realize this need strongly enough to tear down a century of accumulated bias and prejudice. Therefore, when the total communication concept suddenly appeared on the horizon, it came as a very welcome surprise.

*The program is presently at the Taft School.

However, after watching the new philosophy in operation for some years, I have developed a feeling that some of its proponents have probably gone overboard in their enthusiasm, and neglected one or two needs. I am very much aware that speech and speechreading are an integral part of total communication, and I feel that in their surprise and delight at what total communication is accomplishing for little deaf children, their teachers have forgotten that speech and speechreading are very much a foreign language to these youngsters, and that merely using simultaneous communication is not enough for the children to develop maximum oral skills.

I believe that throughout their school years deaf youngsters should get more extensive practice in oral skills than they can get from simultaneous communication alone. Speech and speechreading should be treated as a foreign language, so that at least a class period each day is devoted to oral drill alone, or that it be possible for a hearing teacher to use oral communication alone when teaching a certain subject for a period. Proper attitudes among the children can easily be established by treating the acquisition of oral skills as a delightful game instead of a grim life or death task. These skills can be reinforced by amplification with electronic devices and individual sessions with speech therapists. And, I am certain that the use of manual communication to correct pronunciation and to check speechreading would make the life of the oral teacher much easier and more pleasant.

Preschool and elementary programs for deaf children should be comprehensive enough for them to receive optimum attention and treatment from their teachers. In a proposed plan for the improvement of the education of the deaf by the California Department of Education several years ago, the minimum number of classes in a preschool or elementary program for the deaf was set at seven, and the maximum number of children in each class was determined to be six for the younger ages and seven for the older ages.

Although a larger and more comprehensive elementary program would be more desirable for deaf children, I feel that the
above guidelines are the best possible compromise between the
needs of deaf children for really comprehensive educational
programs (which would necessitate covering much larger areas
and subsequent long-distance busing), and propinquity to their
homes and families for a more normal and healthy environment (that is, *if* their families cooperate by learning to communicate totally with their deaf children).

As is the growing practice in programs for deaf children,
teacher aides should be employed whenever possible. A
thought should also be given to employing at least one deaf
teacher in each program for the younger deaf children, for the
appearance of a deaf adult would be of incalculable benefit to
the children; they would be better able to develop a healthy
self-image and to establish strong rapport with the deaf
teacher. The administrator can easily schedule a rotation of the
classes in order for the children to obtain the necessary instruction and assistance in developing their oral skills from hearing
teachers.

I feel that during their early years, the parents of deaf
children play a very important role in their initial development. Therefore, parent education and counseling should be a
strong part of the program, and the parents should be urged to
develop communicative skills so that there will be no block in
the way of full communication between the parents and their
deaf child. Also, for an ideal family situation, the deaf child's
siblings and other relatives who may share the household
should also learn total communication, and use it all the time in
the presence of the deaf child so that he/she will always feel involved with the family. This way of living will guarantee that
the deaf child will develop normal mental health and emotional stability.

As deaf children approach puberty and adulthood, their
needs begin to change, and it becomes necessary for parents to

gradually let go so that their children can establish their own life and be free to choose friends and career. Young deaf adults' educational needs now begin to grow outside of classroom situations toward extracurricular activities and a satisfying social life.

Therefore, the best secondary program for deaf youngsters seems to be a facility sufficiently large to develop its own extracurricular programs, such as athletics, organizational activities, social affairs, etc. A minimum enrollment of 500 for such a facility does not seem unreasonable, although author James B. Conant has this to say in *The Comprehensive High School: A Second Report to Interested Citizens:*

> I am prepared to maintain that an excellent comprehensive high school can be developed in any school district provided the high school enrolls at least 750 students . . . (p. 2)

Ideally, this facility should be self-contained and full-service so that the deaf students will be able to develop a healthy sense of belonging; they should be able to participate fully in every activity that may be going on and have the opportunity to develop any latent abilities that they may possess. In other words, they should have the chance to compete in a normal manner outside of the classroom without having to contend with the additional handicap of deafness.

Following this line of thought, I cannot approve fragmentary programs for deaf students in regular secondary programs for hearing youngsters. When the deaf students find themselves to be in a small minority, which is different from the large hearing student body, and thus face formidable competition for whatever they may wish to do outside of classes, it is inevitable that their self-image and self-respect will be undermined. They will likely be haunted with a feeling of being different and imperfect, thus developing an inferiority complex for the rest of their lives.

I will be the first to admit that there is validity in the inevitable rebuttal that deaf youngsters will eventually have to

compete with hearing coworkers when they go out in the working world, so why not prepare them by integrating them into a
hearing high school program? My feeling is that adolescent
youngsters need to build a strong and positive self-image first
in an environment where they will have a fair chance to compete, before they are subjected to the unequal competition of
the industrial world.

In a secondary program there should be a greater number of
deaf teachers and also a greater opportunity for qualified deaf
persons to assume administrative and policy-making positions.
The same emphasis on the development of oral skills should be
carried to the secondary program from elementary programs,
and the same opportunities be available to maintain oral skills.
Scheduling can easily be arranged to rotate the deaf youngsters
so that they will have hearing teachers part of the day to provide the necessary assistance with oral skills. Deaf teachers and
administrators should join the others in actively developing
positive attitudes toward the maintenance and practice of
speech and speechreading.

The general feeling seems to be that young deaf people
should have had comprehensive pre-vocational training by the
time they are through with a secondary education, so that their
prime interest should now be to obtain the necessary specialized education and training to get started on a career. Therefore,
aside from a few collegiate programs, post-secondary programs
for deaf students are mainly fragmentary bits of vocationally-
oriented community college programs where supporting services of interpreting and note-taking are provided.

Of the three full four-year collegiate programs available for
deaf students, only Gallaudet College and the National
Technical Institute for the Deaf (NTID) are full-service
institutions. NTID has constructed separate facilities for its
students on the campus of Rochester Institute of Technology,
Rochester, New York.

There is, of course, always the question of preparing the deaf
student for integration into hearing society and more so when

he has to pursue his career among hearing colleagues and supervisors. It is my opinion that when a deaf person is adequately educated, and permitted to build a healthy self-image through participation in activities among his own kind, he is capable of coping with the inevitable pressures and problems of working and communicating with hearing people. It would not be doing him any service to damage his psychological make-up by compelling him to live with and compete with hearing contemporaries in an educational situation; he needs to feel that he is as good as anybody else before he begins to interact with hearing coworkers.

There are various ways in which an educational program can orient the deaf student to interact with hearing persons. Athletic competition with hearing teams is an excellent way; after-game social events, or even occasional parties, which include guests from outside hearing schools should be encouraged. To encourage maximum interaction, it is possible to orient the hearing guests by giving them an opportunity to learn the manual alphabet and maybe a few basic signs before attending these mixed events, and further by providing interpreters at these gatherings to take care of any communication difficulties. At the same time, the deaf students should also be given orientation for interacting with hearing people who may either have failed to learn manual communication or be too bashful to make overtures. The deaf students should be taught to go more than halfway in starting conversations; they should be taught not to be too shy to use whatever speech they may possess, and implement it with gestures or homemade signs if their hearing friends should not know manual communication.

Another way is work-study arrangements, which some educational programs have started. The National Technical Institute for the Deaf has a splendid program in which their deaf students have the opportunity to work in business or industry as part of a work-study plan to gain on-the-job experience while attending NTID at Rochester Institute of

Technology. Thus, they have the opportunity to adjust themselves to the everyday world of work.

The NTID program also provides opportunities for deaf students to integrate with hearing students at Rochester Institute of Technology. Juniors and seniors in upper division collegiate work may enroll in programs offered by RIT with support services such as interpreters, tutors, notetakers and counselors.

7 P.L. 94-142 and Mainstreaming

The passage of Public Law 94-142 (Education for All Handicapped Children Act of 1975) excited probably all handicapped groups except knowledgeable persons in the field of education of deaf children. This includes not only hearing professionals with insight into problems of deafness, but also deaf citizens themselves. Although this public law does not mandate mainstreaming, they have become synonymous to many persons, so in many educational situations mainstreaming handicapped children in regular public schools was the very first step taken.

Deafness constitutes a unique handicap in this setting. There is no problem of physical access to school facilities; indeed deaf children would perhaps be the first handicapped group allowed into schools. But, when it comes down to starting on the educational process itself, appalling difficulties arise. Because deafness is a communicative handicap, not only does the educational process break down, but there are also serious social and psychological stresses placed upon deaf children. This has been very difficult for even the other handicapped groups to understand.

The position statements of the International Association of Parents of the Deaf on Public Law 94-142 and mainstreaming are given below, for they explain very clearly the problems and challenges with which we are faced.

Public Law 94-142:

Public Law 94-142 (Education for All Handicapped Children Act of 1975) guarantees all handicapped children ages 3-21, preschool through grade 12: a free, appropriate public education in the least restrictive environment, due process safeguards, confidentiality of information and nondiscriminatory evaluation. Additionally, PL 94-142 requires the following: public participation in the development of state plans, in-service training for professionals, equal employment opportunities for the handicapped, use of native language in certain situations, elimination of architectural barriers and state advisory panels.

The key accountability measure in PL 94-142 is the Individual Education Program (IEP) which must be developed for each handicapped child by the child's family and school jointly. The IEP which serves as an annual blueprint for the child's educational programming, specifies goals and objectives based on accurate description to the child's current level of educational performance evaluation criteria. Placement of the child and provision of supportive services are determined by the child's basic needs and abilities as documented in the IEP.

Public Law 94-142 is a commendable law; however, problems arise as a result of different interpretations of the law and insufficient understanding of the specific needs of hearing impaired children. The basic intent of PL 94-142 is not simply to mainstream (integration of handicapped children in the least restrictive environment) but to diversify, expand and improve educational opportunities for individual handicapped children.

Parents need to understand their rights under PL 94-142, their child's abilities and needs, and the different educational opportunities available in order to advocate their child's right to the most appropriate educational placement and program. Parents and professionals need to work together as an educational decision making team.

Position:
IAPD supports PL 94-142 and takes the position that parents and professionals should understand fully the intent and provisions of PL 94-142, the ramifications of deafness, and the quality of available programs, in order to ensure that the hearing impaired child is placed and served in an educational environment that will best meet his/her individual needs.

In addition, viable communication and information sharing between the home and the school through the vehicle of the IEP and regular school procedures will facilitate the monitoring of the appropriateness of the child's placement and program.

Mainstreaming:

Current legislation states that "all handicapped children should be taught with non-handicapped children whenever possible" or that handicapped children should be educated in the "least restrictive environment." Legislation of this nature endeavors to implement a concept for the education of handicapped children which is often referred to as "mainstreaming." Although mainstreaming has different definitions, it is generally considered to mean the education of handicapped children among non-handicapped children in a local public school system. The legislation also requires that the needs of the handicapped children be met and that they have services and resources which enable them to compete equally with the non-handicapped child. This later dimension is seldom mentioned but is definitely a part of the concept of "mainstreaming."

This concept is very appealing, but its implementation in present day local public schools will constitute a challenge. If handicapped children are placed in regular classes without appropriate support, they are subjected to blatant discrimination and are almost sure to withdraw or fail. Currently many local and public schools lack needed special services such as qualified diagnostic staff for making the placement of a hearing impaired child, supportive services, trained personnel, necessary amplification equipment and a conducive visual environment, an understanding of total communication which may be essential for communication with students and in many cases both commitment and financial resources required for the education of deaf children.

Parents should be aware of these problems so that their child is not subjected to an educational environment in which he/she has little chance of success.

Position:

It is the position of IAPD to support the best educational programs for hearing impaired children. For some children, placement in regular classrooms will be effective; however, it is necessary for parents to understand that the use of programs in the form of special classes, day schools for the deaf, special schools or residential schools should imply no stigma and is frequently more appropriate.

It is the position of IAPD to focus attention on the achievement and growth of the whole child in the edcuational program first and to consider the proximity of the hearing impaired child to hearing students as desirable but secondary.

Criteria for Mainstreaming:
Some of the criteria to use in deciding if a child should be mainstreamed are as follows:

Child
  Age (within 2 years of peers)
  Maturity
  Self-confidence
  Grade-level functioning
  Ability to adapt
  Communication/language skills
Family
  Support and encouragement
  Communication skills
School
  Teacher attitude and preparation
  Attitude of non-handicapped classmates
  Audio-visual technology
  Curriculum
  Social services and support
  Interpreter services
  Orientation for personnel
  Employment of handicapped professionals
  Special class or resource room consideration
  Types, kinds, ages of children in proposed class
  Success of school graduates/leavers
  Orientation to deafness/sign language classes for staff and hearing students

Public Law 94-142 does not mandate mainstreaming but appropriate educational placement of each handicapped child in the least restrictive environment. However, to the large majority of physically disabled citizens, it means that they would be able to leave special institutions and programs and enjoy equal access to regular public school programs. It is also natural for them to regard the more open and normal atmosphere of public schools as being the ''least restrictive environment.'' If children are so severely physically disabled that they are unable to make progress in such milieu, they are placed in special settings. Therefore, it is evident that people relate mainstreaming failures to special institutions and the term, "most restrictive environment."

With the stigma of failure and the term, "most restrictive environment," automatically connected with special schools, it becomes most difficult for the parents of deaf children to accept the concept that deafness is a unique handicap which affects communication channels rather than physical ability. Deaf students, therefore, require different consideration than the other disabled groups. Because of this, the thinking has to be completely reversed for deaf children—that is, mainstreamed situations are easily the most restricted environment for our special children because they are for most purposes isolated from the regular public school population; and special schools for them are the least restricted environment, where everybody is specially trained to communicate and work with deaf children. Indeed, these special facilities may be regarded as miniature communities where deaf children can interact in a very normal manner and thereby achieve the usual rate of growth and maturity.

This fact has been so little understood by legislatures and courts that decisions have been made which are inimical to the best interests of deaf children. Dr. Mervin D. Garretson, special assistant to the President of Gallaudet College, presented testimony at a hearing questioning the functions of a state school for the deaf. Below is a reproduction of his paper, entitled "The Deaf Child and the Unwritten Curriculum," from *The Deaf American* which was a direct outgrowth of that testimony. I am including it because I feel that it describes the problem in an extremely lucid manner.

> Today Public Law 94-142 is the acknowledged law of the land. It includes amendments to P.L. 93-380 which provided the base for many of the current statutes and special education codes among

our states. The new law provides for a variety of school settings which include public residential schools, with emphasis on the concept of least restrictive environment commensurate with the unique needs of each handicapped child. It was never the intent of this legislation to discriminate against any specific handicapped group. Through successive drafts of the federal regulations interpreting the law, the original hierarchy of school settings has undergone modification to become a range of options selected in accordance with the overall educational needs of each individual child. Because the educative process in regular public schools is primarily auditory-based, a well-staffed day school or a residential school frequently is the most conducive to an appropriate educational program for the deaf child, and therefore his/her *least* restrictive alternative.

P.L. 94-142 is rooted in three basic guarantees or rights. Its stated purpose is (1) to assure that all handicapped children have available to them a free, appropriate public education and related services to meet their unique needs. It is important that we underscore *free, appropriate,* and *related services.* (2) The second purpose is to assure that the rights of handicapped children and their parents are protected, and (3) to assure the effectiveness of efforts to educate handicapped children.

For a number of reasons, including the low incidence handicap of deafness, two out of every one thousand, and because of the subtle implications of hearing impairment and the ever-present spectre of communication barriers, invariably it is the day or residential school which provides an appropriate, quality program in terms of homogenous grouping, adequate peer interaction, trained teachers, professional supervision, appropriate curriculum, relevant visual materials and equipment, a communicating environment, and comprehensive supportive serivces. Very few, if any, local programs are able to justify all of these requisite resources. The observation might be made that the due process sections of this landmark legislation provide for legal challenge of any halfbaked program that does not completely meet the needs of each handicapped child.

Before approaching the report itself, it may be helpful to examine some of the parameters of general learning, both within and peripheral to the classroom and their relevance to hearing loss and to community perspectives. It is my belief that these considerations are germane to the issue before us today, particularly with regard to special education practitioners who exhibit the usual naivete about gut-level realities of deafness.

For some time it has been my feeling that what I characterize as "the unwritten curriculum" has been one of the most overlooked aspects of the total education picture—an extension of the non-schooling process of crucial significance in the life of the deaf child with his communication handicap. The residential-day school provides the needed totality of experience, serves as the educational community, the social system, if you will, which is so necessary during the formative years for the development of self-concept and human relationships which carry over into adult life.

First, let's look at the average year in the daily living of a normal school-age student—that is, a full 365 days multiplied by 24, which gives us a total of 8,760 hours. Since most school systems appear to operate on a 180-day school year, this adds up to 720 hours of actual classroom time out of the 8,760—or a mere 8 percent. What happens to the other 92 percent of the year when the child is not in school?

It is possible to do some fairly close estimating. From information that the average child spends a total of 50 hours a week in front of the television set, and by allowing for 8 hours of sleep, time for meals and snacks, estimating periods utilized for play, movies, visiting, shopping, personal hygiene, travel, and other miscellaneous activities we are able to distribute a child's 8,760 hours during a normal year as follows:

2,600 hours, viewing television

2,920 hours, sleeping or napping

1,095 hours, eating (meals and snacks)

1,425 hours, miscellaneous

720 hours, at school

From this we may make a number of immediate observations: (1) A child spends more time watching TV than in school; (2) more time sleeping than in school; (3) more time eating than in school; (4) more time in miscellaneous activities than in school. The child's non-schooling hours are more than 11 times those spent in the classroom.

One conclusion we arrive at is that the average hearing child receives the bulk of his educational or learning experience during the 92 percent of the time he is not in a regular classroom situation. On the other hand, this conclusion is rarely true for the deaf child unless a number of extremely vital conditions are met, understood, and planned for—within what we understand as the unwritten curriculum.

Curriculum as we understand it is actually limited to learnings that are developed through schooling. Objectives of a curriculum generally revolve around human need goals, the intellectual, social, physical, and emotional well-being of an individual. P.L. 94-142 correctly perceives educational programming as encompassing much more than mere academics. In addition to the basic R's and other subject-matter knowledge, an educational plan means developing social, psychomotor, self-help, and communication skills. Education includes acquiring adaptive ability, emotional maturity, prevocational training, and skills at daily living activities. Provision is made for learning group participation techniques, understanding and interpretation of values, opportunities for exercising leadership, learning how to learn on one's own, developing cope-ability. Education aims toward a healthy self-concept for each child—in short, development of the whole person.

The unwritten curriculum refers to all of those activities, planned and unplanned, which I perceive as nonschooling aspects of learning. Accepted as a matter of course by educators in general since it's practically automatic for normally hearing children, the label exists for me only in relationship to deafness. An approximate synonymous term may be "incidental learning," but I believe the adjective suggests a deceptive and simplistic perception of what is a highly significant aspect of the deaf child's educational experience.

What is the learning milieu of the average child with normal hearing aside from time spent in school? Many of us with hearing children know that our kids reached a fairly sophisticated understanding of English syntax, use of idiom, and a full-blown vocabulary before they ever set foot inside a school or formal classroom. During these early prekindergarten years they also picked up counting, elements of set theory and other mathematical concepts (without their technical names, of course),—they learned a great deal of history and geography from television, radio, peer and adult conversations. They absorbed facts and understandings about social codes and attitudes (psychology), health habits and games (physical education), and countless other things that today may have fancy names in some curriculum shops. Children and youth, provided there is adequate communication, do tend to learn more by example than by precept; more from the world as it is than through admonition, lecturing, or demonstration.

The hearing child's total education, both the written and un-written curriculum is readily accessible—particularly the latter, in-fluenced as it is by innumerable "teachers" such as the mass media (newspapers, magazines, TV, radio), the home, the street, novels and other books, self-instructional materials and what one learns from his peer group or on the job. And with normal hearing the child is able to utilize his language foundation to expand his educa-tion and to extend his learning horizons both in and out of school.

Ivan Illich of the Cuernavaca think-tank has said that "most people when pressed to specify how they acquired what they know and value will readily admit that they learned it more often outside than inside school. Their knowledge of facts, their understanding of life and work came to them from friendship or love, while view-ing TV, or while reading, from examples of peers or the challenge of a street encounter."

The noted Amherst scholar and professor Henry Steele Com-mager in his address at the 1974 Atlantic City convention of the American Association of School Administrators made the observa-tion that "it is, after all, the community which performs the major job of education, not the schools; performs through a hundred miscellaneous institutions from family to farm, from government to playing field, from churches to labor unions, from newspapers and journals to comics and radio, and above all, television."

So, for the deaf child, where is the community? Nine times out of 10 the hearing community is a physical presence but a mental blankness. That is where the naivete comes in. Deafness is invisi-ble and people rarely see beyond the surface. Of partial help is a family which has adopted total communication so that the deaf child becomes part of the environment, coupled with a large residential or day school with a variety of peer contacts and adults who know and use communication, including utilization in and out of class of captioned films, and other visuals, interpreters, and all sorts of reinforcement. While these positives will not cover the full 92 percent of the unwritten curriculum, they will go a long way in assisting the child during his early, crucial years to build the foundations upon which he can further his education and use it as a springboard to move confidently into the greater world beyond childhood.

Another example of the full meaning of communication as un-consciously assumed by the hearing child came to me not long ago in an article in the *Washington Post*. Printed several weeks ago, this news item reported that students in Columbus, Ohio, were returning to school after the energy shortage had closed 140 public schools in that area for a full month. Upon returning to the classrooms the students were almost unanimous in stating that they had learned a great deal more during that month than they would have in school. During this enforced vacation created by a lack of natural gas to heat their schools, the kids learned from educational features published in the two daily newspapers, from three commercial TV stations and a radio station which provided classroom broadcasts by teachers, and from expanded programming by the educational radio outlet. The business community opened wide its doors. Classes were held in beer parlors, pizza cafes, billiard halls, and corporate board rooms. Tours were conducted through foundries, glass factories, banks, and insurance offices—exposing the students to a side of business normally not open to them. For the occasional deaf student mainstreamed here and there in these 140 public schools, all of this was practically a total loss. Did the teachers on the radio and television use sign language? Were interpreters provided on the tours and by the business community? Most likely not. For the hearing impaired child the unwritten curriculum simply did not exist.

Let's look again at the regular public school setting, at the four hours or so a child is in class each school day. An inestimable amount of peripheral learning is supplementing the formal curriculum in-between classes, at the library or media center, during recess, at lunchtime, during physical education, choir practice, independent artwork and laboratory period time, and of course the endless after-school activities: intramural and varsity athletics, student body government functions and meetings, and all of the extracurricular clubs, debate, French, drama, Spanish, chess, and so on. Generally the deaf child tags along as a wallflower, a silent member of the crowd, present and yet absent, a second-class participant with latent leadership abilities undeveloped and dormant without much of a chance to contribute. At an extreme he is but a stifled shape of lifeless clay—"helpless piece of the game he plays/Upon the chequer-board of nights and days."

Many departments of education continue not to understand the unique and subtle disability of hearing loss which leads to a highly complicated communication handicap. In making omnibus state plans for all handicapped children, generalizing over a wide range of disparate disabilities, what needs to be taken into account is the fact that in a regular public school situation other handicapped children such as the blind and the orthopedically handicapped are able to—

1. hear the teacher
2. hear their classmates in front, behind, and all around them
3. hear and participate in class discussions
4. hear the educational film presented in class
5. hear the principal over the public address system
6. hear the visiting speaker invited for that period
7. hear the guide on the class field trip
8. hear the radio or television program assigned to the class
9. hear the exchange of friendly chit-chat at recess
10. hear the quick peer interaction when going down the hall between classes
11. hear the news and gossip during lunch hour
12. hear the "sum up" on the walk home at day's end
13. hear the debates during student body government meetings
14. hear all of the other countless items that come almost as if by osmosis and of which every one is practically unaware

The simple fact is that the deaf child does not hear.

Hearing-impairment tends to project a surface invisibility (most people internalize only what they see, like the exposed tip of an iceberg, for example). This superficial perception of deafness may account for the a priori assumption that a local school program is appropriate for deaf children and somehow will meet all of their needs. Actually, the basic thrust in regular public school settings is one of refinement and increment of already existing knowledges, information banks, and language skills within a hearing-structured classroom, under a hearing-structured relationship, and encompassed by a hearing-structured environment.

Careful analysis of the foregoing parmeters should suggest that a state educational plan for deaf children be developed around their genuine educational needs rather than from the standpoint of organizational expediency.

Economic feasibility is another question which needs scrutiny. This must be viewed within the context of low-incidence and homogenous grouping, and also as to whether a local education district may realistically justify the tremendous cost of maintaining an adequate program for only a few students. Pro-rata cost of supportive services will be exorbitant: speech pathologist, audiologist/auditory training specialist, trained counselor of the deaf, psychological services, interpreter-tutors, special training for regular teachers, captioned educational films, and other costly media equipment—all of which is pretty much available right now at residential/day schools. Most important, perhaps, is the fact that the residential school provides direct round-the-clock teaching. At this juncture we might note that a recent study at the National Technical Institute for the Deaf at Rochester Institute of Technology reveals that deaf students retain more from direct total-communication instruction than through third-party interpreters.

On the other side of the coin, not to be overlooked is the price of mainstreaming to the LEA's and their non-deaf children in terms of time, energy, and training expended on regular school instruction and its resources. What of the cost of time and attention diverted from the 25 to 30 hearing children in each classrooms which will be necessary for adequate service to each small group of communicatively handicapped children? I have just learned recently of a disturbing trend at the Maryland School for the Deaf which probably represents an index of what is happening in other states. Each year the school has been admitting increasing number of hearing impaired children 10 years of age or older who have developed learning and emotional problems in regular public schools. The Maryland School reports that it is saddled with the formidable task of remediation, counseling, and redirection of these children. Of newly enrolled children in the Maryland School in 1973, 31 percent were transfers from public schools; in 1974, 36 percent; in 1975, 56 percent, and in 1976, they received a full 61 percent as educational failures resulting from misconceived placement.

Three "key imperatives" for state programming in the area of hearing-impairment have been identified by Barry L. Griffing, assistant superintendent of public instruction and assistant director of the California Office of Special Education:

1) A state must assure itself that every deaf child, youth, and adult has access to an educational opportunity of adequate scope and quality.

2) A state, having diversity in population and needs, must utilize all available resources or make new ones to meet the range of needs of deaf individuals.

3) A state must organize its educational opportunity resources for

the deaf to create a reasonable relationship of responsibility among those managing the resources.

One might envision a continuation of present programs with qualitiative modification as needed, and an expanded role in such components as:

1) Serve as a part of every LEA/ISD in each state as a viable and least restrictive alternative for deaf children should their IEP so indicate;

2) Develop and implement a program for the gifted deaf children of the state as well as for the multiply handicapped;

3) Serve as a comprehensive demonstration/resource/training center for other programs in the state;

4) Develop early childhood and parent programs;

5) Develop a career planning model;

6) Make available its facilities and resources as a community and continuing education center during afterschool hours, and

7) Experiment with reverse and partial mainstreaming with selected students.

Finally, I am deeply concerned that out of the maze of jurisdictional concerns, operational and organizational logistics, statutes and special education codes, questionable approaches to economics and other dimensions of the Pandora's box, somehow the deaf child has become lost. We have all forest and no trees. The child is dehumanized into a statistic, a piece of movable data. Should mainstreaming continue to be an end in itself, and should the residential school be eliminated as a desirable option for the normal deaf children of each state, I fear that legal and moral laws will be violated, but more than this, I fear that somewhere, somehow, in this country little deaf children will be educationally, vocationally, and emotionally mutilated. This must not happen.

I can only say, "Amen!" to this. Let every concerned person sit up and take notice of the many pitfalls involved in mainstreaming deaf children in regular public school programs so that a new generation of educational failures may not come forth to become social and economic burdens on society, not to mention the great damage done to the mental health of these deaf individuals by turning them out to be frustrated and un-fulfilled adults.

8 The Deaf Adult

Types of Deaf Adults

Deaf adults cannot be stereotyped; they are essentially human beings with normal faculties, abilities, and weaknesses except for a deficient sense of hearing. However, because of the nature of the etiology of deafness, a larger proportion of deaf people than hearing have additional handicaps.

On the other hand, deaf adults possess certain qualities common to them because of the things that they have missed during their growth and development due to their loss of hearing and communicative difficulties.

It may be helpful if I attempt to portray the various kinds of deaf adults there are in an average community of deaf people. There seem to be three main factors influencing the development of deaf children into adults: (1) the degree and kind of deafness, (2) the amount of native intelligence, and (3) the environmental components, which include education, family, and community.

If we examine the three factors, we find that two of them are not controllable. The miracle of modern medicine has reduced the incidence of deafness from various illnesses later in life, such as measles, scarlet fever, etc. At the same time it has contributed toward a greater rate of survival among defective infants. Therefore, the incidence of deafness has shifted from post-lingual years toward pre-lingual years, and the involvement of additional handicaps is greater now.

The only controllable factor seems to be the deaf adult's environmental effects which include the education that he has received. As has been said in the chapter on traditional educational methods, the results have been highly unsatisfactory.

Moreover, his family members and the people in his immediate community have been more likely than not exposed to the prevailing dominance of oralism, which has been enforced by great amounts of propaganda and a great number of pseudo-authorities on deafness. They may have been thereby persuaded to confine their communication with the deaf person to the highly restrictive and impeditive oral means. Thus, we see a deaf adult who has been handicapped and impeded in more ways than merely his deafness.

These three factors should be kept in mind when we scrutinize deaf adults and their communities. There are not two communities of deaf people which are alike; they range from the intellectual and sophisticated community which grew around Gallaudet College, a four-year liberal arts college for the deaf in Washington, D.C., to small and naive rural communities. However, we may find discernable patterns of deaf persons in these communities.

Adventitiously deaf adults—These persons lost their hearing after they had acquired language and speech, so they are probably the "elite" among deaf people. They have the best language, and are frequently asked by the others to help them with letters, messages, etc. Since most of them still have some usable language, they are usually the spokespersons for the community. These people, on the average, lost their hearing between the ages of five and 12, and completed their education in programs for the deaf, where they became acquainted with other deaf students and were introduced into their community. Persons who lose their hearing at ages older than 12 are more likely to remain with their former hearing friends, and struggle along with the help of hearing aids and speechreading practice, for there are very few of those people who have joined the community of deaf adults.

Pre-lingually deaf adults who come from deaf families—On the whole, these persons are about on a par with those who are post-lingually deaf, for they had early communication, and therefore are more likely to have better than average language, although they may have no usable speech. Since they have encountered practically no frustrations because of their deafness, they are more outgoing and at ease with other deaf persons. They also frequently become the leaders in the deaf community.

Other pre-lingually deaf adults—They are the bulk of the deaf community. They come from hearing families who have had trouble communicating with them when they were little. Consequently, for the most part, they have difficulties with expressing themselves in English. Their early deafness has generally prevented them from developing speech as good as that of the adventitiously deaf. They have had more frustrations than the deaf adults in the first two groups, so they, for the most part, lack aggressiveness and self-confidence.

Low-verbal deaf adults—These adults have missed a great deal of education that they should have received for various reasons, so they are almost illiterate. They may be able to sign their own names, and write simple sentences, phrases, or words, but certainly, not long or involved sentences; nor can they read anything but simple English constructions. They are able to express themselves with exaggerated signs, maybe mixed with homemade pantomime. There are various reasons for their retardation: they might have been slow learners; oral failures who were kept in oral programs until they were too old to continue, went to residential schools too late to get any real help, or were kept in public schools to stagnate; or they may be members of culturally deprived families.

Products of oral programs—Many products of oral schools have found their lives to be more rewarding when they learned manual communication and joined the community of deaf adults. They were soon signing and fingerspelling among the best of the manual deaf adults, but they are for the most part easy to distinguish because their oral schooling has left its mark on them, such as habitually mouthing when signing.

Products of public schools—Another category is those who went through regular public school programs without the benefit of interpreting services. If they succeeded at their schoolwork, I am inclined to suspect that they have extraordinary abilities, are mildly or moderately hard of hearing, or were deafened later in life. If they are average or less in their ability, they are very likely to get very little from their public school programs—and what is worse, to have developed a lifelong habit of inattentiveness while maintaining an alert look for their teachers' benefit. They have developed various strategems to meet and satisfy life's various demands without alerting concerned persons, such as their own parents, to their shortcomings. Many of these persons are low verbal.

Uneducated deaf adults—We must not overlook those deaf adults who have had very few years of schooling or none at all, and are, therefore, uneducated for practical purposes. When we consider that they have no means of communication on top of their lack of education, then we must realize that they are indeed at the very bottom stratum of the deaf community, and, therefore, are objects of pity and charity. However, there are many who have been so self-reliant that they have managed to obtain an education, after a fashion by themselves. These deaf adults have turned out to be hard-working and useful deaf citizens, although they are by necessity confined to either farming or menial work.

Deafened adults—There are individuals who lost their hearing after they were well through their educational programs, probably due to illness, injury, war wounds, or to the debilitating effects of old age. Although they are just as deaf as the deaf adults under consideration, they are in an entirely different category. They have developed as hearing persons, and have all the attributes possessed by individuals without any loss of hearing. Their late deafness does not suddenly change their make-up; in fact, the handicap does not take anything away from them except their hearing. Therefore, their problems are entirely different; they have normal speech but probably have a much greater need for hearing aids to activate an already well-developed auditory sense. In addition to this need, they require an extensive training in speechreading in order to carry on the same communication modes they have been using for so long.

They probably number more than the deaf under scrutiny here, but very few of these persons have been both motivated and able to make the big jump into the community of the deaf as we know it. They usually follow one of two courses of action, again depending upon the many and various factors involved in their loss of hearing: either continue in the same environment with the same circle of acquaintances with the help of a hearing aid and an acquired skill in speechreading; or gradually withdraw from their former friends into a lonely existence or into a new circle of friends who are similarly afflicted. Even though deaf, they are hearing persons in mind and spirit, and therefore leagues away from those who have been deaf since an early age.

The few representatives of this group who have accomplished the large adjustment to become members of our deaf community usually take advantage of their attainments to achieve leadership roles. These persons, together with others who were deafened after they had acquired speech, were the bellwethers who accomplished the breakthrough of the deaf into decision and policy-making positions.

Hard of hearing adults—We must not forget another group of hearing impaired persons—the hard of hearing. It is very difficult to draw a line between them and the deaf as there are many who are borderline cases. The hard of hearing have residual hearing which is functional; in other words, they are able to make sense out of what they hear. This has a great implication in their education and development. With amplification by hearing aids they are usually able to acheive at a more normal pace, and are usually more acceptable to the hearing community. If they choose to join the deaf community, they often become leaders who are accepted by both the hearing and deaf community.

There is a humorous aspect of this acceptance of deaf adults with good speech by the hearing community. There are deaf adults who have mediocre speech which is usually difficult for their hearing acquaintances to understand. These persons have found that if they put on hearing aids, even though of no actual benefit to them they would find themselves better understood by strangers. Apparently the very appearance of hearing aids has a beneficial psychological effect upon the listening ability of the hearing strangers. There have also been instances where a hearing person was able to follow a deaf person's speech quite well until he discovered that the latter was deaf. Then, he would be unable to understand a single word!

There are many other factors besides deafness and education which contribute to the make-up of deaf adults, such as additional handicaps, racial problems, and religious persuasions. For example, before the southern schools for the deaf were integrated, black deaf children had to be content with inferior educational programs which turned them out as inferior deaf adults. Chicano and American Indian deaf students did not have integration problems, but like the blacks, they did not receive special treatment to provide for their different cultures and languages, nor for the training of their parents and teachers.

A Psychological Perspective
It is difficult to paint you a picture of deafness, for I have been deaf all my life, and I have no frame of reference against which to compare my deafness. However, other deaf friends have occasionally described their feelings about deafness when it occurred later in life. As a general rule, the later you become deaf, the harder the adjustment to the handicap. I have seen some say how they missed listening to music, participating fully in the activities of their old gang of hearing friends, etc.

I would like to digress to say that I have noticed a strange phenomenon about the attitudes of deaf adults toward hearing people. Deaf adults who were children of deaf parents seem to regard hearing persons a little differently from those who had hearing parents. Deaf children of deaf parents have never had frustrations because they had full communication and understanding parents all their life, while the others must have had bad moments during their lives, when their hearing parents discovered their deafness and found it to be a problem living and communicating with their deaf children; their expressions and utterances showing grief, disappointment, and impatience must have been obvious to the deaf youngsters. Such displays must have been very traumatic to the deaf children's pride, self-satisfaction, and self-image. And, they must have become adjusted to a feeling of inferiority, which deaf children of deaf parents do not usually develop. Therefore, the latter are quicker to notice and resent any show of superiority or paternalism by hearing people than the former. Deaf adults with hearing parents seem to expect, and accept better the superior attitude of hearing persons.

However, all deaf adults are subject to the same frustrations when they attempt to go about the daily business of living. For instance, Alexander Graham Bell, the father of oralism, is in our bad graces not only because he began the frustrating and impeditive philosophy of oralism in the education of deaf children, but also because he invented the telephone! Instead of being the convenience that it is for hearing persons, it is one more stumbling block in deaf adults' aspirations for advancement in their jobs. The telephone has been offered more often than anything else as an excuse for not promoting deserving deaf employees; their inability to answer the phone has ruined many deaf workers' hopes for supervisory positions.

In the appendix are excellent mental pictures of deafness, which are painted by three deaf educators: Shanny Mow, Roy Holcomb, and Lawrence Newman. These articles should make you *feel* deafness and help you to build an empathy for deaf people.

Before we begin to consider the psyche of the deaf adult, we should consider the factors which contribute to the deaf person's unique mental outlook. The first factor to think about is the fact that deaf persons constitute a minority group. Therefore, they are subject to the same problems that other minority groups face: the demand that the minority people come up to the expectations of the majority, and majority's utter disregard for the real needs of the minority group; and in addition the preconceived opinions, the prejudices, the power structure, the self-perpetuation, the superiority complex (paternalism), and the authority held by the members of the majority over the minority segment. The majority also has the melting pot, or manifest destiny concept of minority group persons—that all of them have to be the same. Thus, the Indians have their "white fathers;" the blacks, their "whiteys;" the Chicanos, their "gringos;" and the deaf, their "hearies." Any attempt for self-betterment by a minority group is therefore contravened by some of the majority group's determination to maintain the *status quo*.

The second factor is that the very nature of the handicap cuts off the ordinary channels of communication between the deaf and their environment. They are forced by their circumstances to live in isolation unless the others make a determined effort to establish substitute forms of communication that are close to if not as effective as the usual modes of communication: hearing and speech. Unfortunately, the dynamics of minority groups are such that until very recently the majority group of hearing educators has determinedly stuck to its preconceived idea that oralism, or rather, "visible speech and hearing," should be the only mode of communication to be encouraged. And, the minority group of the deaf has had to be content with this partial and imperfect communication, which has impeded the normal input of background information with which the deaf child would have been better able to interact in order to benefit from the full process of education. Thus, this lack of background is taking a terrible toll of deaf persons' chances for a full and optimum development into happy, well-adjusted, and self-sufficient citizens.

Characteristics of Deaf Adults
Since the hearing impaired have had to contend not only with their handicap, but also with other common hindrances, they have developed identifiable characteristics. (Again, other variables come into this consideration to qualify these characteristics so that the following attributes may not apply equally well to each deaf individual.)

Perhaps the first characteristic to be noticed in a deaf adult is his *substandard language ability*. This is no measure at all of his native intelligence. When you consider the fact that the average deaf infant, like all other babies, is born with a clean slate for a mind and is additionally handicapped by the imperfect, faltering, and thwarting aspects of pure oral communication, you must marvel that the deaf person has managed to acquire any language at all during his development!

Recent research has confirmed what deaf adults have long known—that intelligance has absolutely no correlation with speech and speechreading competence. The implication is obvious that language and oral skills can be taught and learned separately.

However, the unfortunate fact remains that the deaf adult has characteristic difficulties in expressing him/herself in acceptable English. A deaf person has trouble distinguishing between active and passive voices and therefore may appear accusing in his/her statements, when, in fact, he/she is merely telling something about himself. A deaf person is usually unable to remember the different forms of a particular root word to show the different parts of speech, so that many words may appear to be out of context. Adjectives may follow nouns, *a la* the romance languages. He/She has appalling difficulties with the use of articles. Such language deficiencies may be listed *ad infinitum.*

This regrettable fact is but another stumbling block in the average deaf adult's communication with his/her milieu. Thus, a vicious circle was started when a deaf child's informal communication was arbitrarily narrowed to a single means, and more so when this pathway was limited to employing the child's deficient organs, rather than bringing into play his other and intact senses. This lack of lucid communication in turn led to the child's increasing language difficulties. The cost of unclear communication is appalling to the deaf child's emotional make-up, leading to deviant behavior and adjustment problems. *It remains for an employer and other significant people in the deaf person's life to realize the material fact that one's language ability does not reflect the amount of one's intelligence at all. It is a common thing to find the deaf adult to be a far superior worker to another person who may possess much better language ability and/or speech and speechreading talents.*

The language difficulties of average deaf adults are reflected in their reading ability. Their level of reading is way below that of the average hearing adult. Since communication has been very limited, his/her understanding has also been limited to concrete concepts. Unless his/her communication becomes rich enough to start to be flexible with the use and meaning of words employed, the deaf adult cannot begin to comprehend the more abstract concepts. Without this advanced understanding, he cannot begin to appreciate the play on words that constitute the standard brand of humor. Lacking this imagination, the average adult is therefore limited to the more earthy and concrete forms of humor.

This, however, is more of a problem than just a lack of cultured humor. The average deaf adult has difficulty comprehending subtleties in language construction, such as idioms, allegories, metaphors, similes, euphemisms, ironies, and other figures of speech.

Because of the weakness mentioned above, the underachieving deaf adult has very shallow ideas of what constitute the pleasures in life; he/she has no concept nor appreciation of the additional pleasures that are obtained by unlocking the treasure chest of classical literature, the various art and craft forms, the diversity of foreign cultures, or the flights of imagination which are created by observing the latest discoveries in science. Therefore, this deaf person is easily satisfied with common surface pleasures which are available: sporting contests, boating, camping, etc. Because of this complacence, and unpleasant experiences with the traditional schooling methods, the average deaf person is not usually interested in further education, such as that offered in adult programs, unless sure that he/she will derive immediate concrete benefits from spending time in adult education classes. Culture, as it is commonly conceived, is foreign to the shortchanged deaf adult.

Because of their communicative handicap, average deaf persons have a tenuous relationship with their general environment. They miss a lot of what is going on around them, and do not immediately become aware of the continuing changes in current styles, fads, modes, or philosophy. From my years of experience with the deaf, I have come to the conclusion that the average deaf adult, even at college level, is approximately two years behind the current trends. For instance, the drug problem among the deaf did not peak until approximately two years after the problem became acute in the hearing world. Similarly, waves of succeeding fads did not peak in the deaf community until a like lag in time had passed.

This lag is evident among young deaf children; they seem to mature mentally slower than they do physically. In many cases this immaturity is carried over into their adulthood because a communicative barrier continues to exist between them and the outside world. They do not speak clearly enough to be understood, they do not get more than a fraction of what they read on the lips, they are unable to comprehend everything that is printed in the daily paper, and they do not have sufficient language to express their thoughts and wants.

It is no wonder that the average deaf adult is often considerably less mature in certain respects than his/her counterpart in the hearing world. The implications of this fact are many. Perhaps the most notable point to be considered is that the deaf adult has extremely short range goals; he/she is much more interested in immediate wants and needs than in any possible benefits in the future. This probably also accounts for the shallowness and complacence frequently found, and explains why civic organizations, such as the National Association of the Deaf and the state associations, have such a hard time recruiting not only membership but also the interest of deaf adults, while recreational groups like the American Athletic Association of the Deaf, the regional bowling and golfing groups, and the local clubs have a much easier time of it.

The deaf adult is also slow in developing an understanding of responsibilities and privileges as an employee, a member of the community, a taxpayer, and a citizen of the United States. Socially immature, the deaf person frequently commits blunders which try the hearing public's tolerance toward him/her. Family isolation, the hesitation of the residential school to "work" him/her, and the failure of the average school program to alert him/her to responsiblities, have contributed toward a "gimme" attitude. Everything has come to the deaf individual without his having to reckon for it, so the deaf adult has grown to take for granted that anything is his/hers for the asking, and that anybody will do his/her bidding. This sorry attitude is due to the hearing majority's failure to be aware that a correct attitude is developed only through everyday, casual participation in familial and community activities, and that such a development is made possible only by free and easy communication both ways. This lack of communication and subsequent understanding and acceptance by the deaf individual is carried over into jobs and activities as a citizen. Therefore, a young deaf person frequently creates a bad reputation for tardiness and failure to report absences in advance, as well as taking Dutch leaves from the job.

There is an angle to this that hearing persons may not be aware of. The difficulty that many deaf adults have to overcome is to "report in" to their employers when they become ill, or when they should be suddenly called away. The dilemna is how they should get the message sent; it is common that their landladies or neighbors have become adverse to making phone calls for them, so they frequently find themselves without a way of letting their bosses know, especially when they are too sick to venture outside.

Therefore, there might have been mitigating reasons for deaf adults' failures to do what they should have done while on the job. It is often through such bitter experiences as being docked or fired because of unexplained absences that deaf adults finally develop an awareness of responsibility and try even harder. Some attempts have been made to inform and instruct young deaf adults about their accountability toward their employers and other things germane to their future vocation. However, these formal courses can never fully take the place of practical observations and experiences which deaf adults have missed due to their communicative handicap.

For the same reasons deaf adults are usually unaware of the public services which are available to them, such as unemployment benefits, legal aid for the indigent, welfare benefits, homes for unwed mothers, planned parenthood agencies, crippled children's services, etc. Most of the time the social workers' concern for unfortunate people who need help does not encompass deaf people. They either hesitate or dislike to assume the burden of establishing communication with them, therefore leaving them in limbo, outside of their areas of concern. Hence, we find deaf adults living a very meager existence, unaware that the needed help is theirs only for the asking. There is a growing number of agencies which help bridge the communication gap for the deaf by counseling them and referring them to proper public agencies with interpreters if needed.

It has been stated previously that deaf persons' inability to hear and monitor their own speech is responsible for the fact that their speech is never normal. This inability to hear their own sounds also has some ramifications. Deaf adults have been known to have an unnecessarily heavy walk which bothers neighbors if they live in a multi-dwelling unit. They may also shuffle their feet. It is not uncommon that they leave water running, or their automobile engine running, with fatal consequences in several known cases. Deaf persons' conversations are frequently accompanied by weird vocal sounds—grunts, groans, whistles, or yells. When deep in reverie, they sometimes emit a humming sound or low grunts. At meal times they may unconsciously create unpleasant noises by dropping silver, scraping the plate with a fork, chewing too loudly, or pushing the chair back abruptly so that the legs make a scraping sound. The deaf individual's laughter or giggle is frequently uninhibited, to the wonder and alarm of the hearing people in the immediate vicinity.

Profoundly deaf adults who were unpleasantly involved with oralism when they were younger—that is, those who had anxious parents putting pressures on them to go through an oral program, with scant success—usually develop bad hang-ups about anything connected with oralism. They shy away from oral deaf adults; they make derogatory remarks about speech and speechreading training. They have a very negative attitude toward audiologists and educators espousing pure oral methods. Deaf persons with employable oral skills usually have some difficulty being accepted by the others with no oral skills unless they successfully belittle their own oral skills.

That deaf adults are highly verbal does not necessarily mean that they are any more intelligent than the less verbal persons; it may mean that they have had better breaks, such as having deaf parents or understanding hearing parents, or being in a favorable educational climate. A tragic aspect of deafness is that because of the methods dispute and inadequate education programs, in many cases, the native intelligence of deaf children is never fully exploited. Therefore, the success stories of educational programs practicing oralism should be scrutinized carefully, for their students go through a selective process, with failures from these programs being sent to residential schools.

The better educated deaf adults on the whole appreciate the value of oral skills more than do the less educated adults. They go into vocations or professions where oral skills become highly useful. Therefore, hard of hearing or deafened adults who indubitably possess more natural and understandable speech are more likely to be accepted by the hearing community than the others.

Most of the leaders of the deaf community, as mentioned before in this chapter, come from this group. However, there are a few instances of non-speaking deaf adults assuming administrative positions lately. It is to be hoped that more of these adults will be accepted into policy- and decision-making positions, for they probably more truly represent the average deaf adults.

An unfortunate consequence of the above, together with the natural result of growing up in a hearing family and being indoctrinated with the greatness and indispensibility of a possession of oral skills, is that some hard of hearing and deafened adults feel themselves to be a notch above the deaf adults who may not be able to speak, no matter how intelligent they may be.

In fact, a pecking order according to the degree of the usability of their oral skills is frequently perceivable among these deaf leaders. Since I do not possess usable speech nor read lips readily, I have been a victim of this attitude many times. These deaf standard-bearers seem to feel that the possession of acceptable oral skills more than make up for any deficiency in other skills, and, at the other extreme, that a want of speech or lipreading ability automatically disqualifies deaf adults from certain roles or responsibilities, even though they may otherwise possess all the qualifications. I may even go on to say that many hearing educators share this viewpoint. As a consequence, the hearing public get to see or deal with deaf leaders who are not truly representative of the great bulk of average deaf adults.

After years of being victims of faulty communication with family and school personnel with consequent misunderstanding and frustrations, young deaf adults are usually happy and anxious to join the society of their own kind. There they can throw off the shackles of halting communication and become fully participating members of the community of the deaf where communication is free and easy.

This fact has been very difficult for their hearing friends to accept.

> A well-known hard of hearing principal of a midwestern school for the deaf finally got tired of attending meetings where hearing administrators continually discussed their concern about ''integrating'' their deaf children into the hearing society. He broke into such a discussion to ask, ''What's so great about the hearing society?'' It would be amusing to observe the dumbfounded expressions of the hearing persons!

This is probably the best expression of how average deaf adults feel; they do not have the slightest desire to ''integrate'' into the hearing community, not only because communication is so difficult and frustrating, but also because their own culture is very attractive to them. Deaf adults can develop a sense of belonging only when they are with their own kind, and there deaf persons prefer to be, knowing that deaf people can belong only to the fringe of a hearing community.

This is, then, a call for public understanding of how members of minority groups interact and feel; the realistic approach would be more tolerance than actual acceptance.

In the appendix is an interesting transcript of a panel discussion by average deaf adults giving their viewpoints on being deaf in today's world.

9 The Community of the Deaf

A Portrayal

Some hearing educators have condescendingly referred to the adult deaf community as "the deaf ghetto," "the deaf subculture," and other uncomplimentary names. Perhaps the best rebuttal would be the National Association of the Deaf's 1972 convention which was held in one of the top hotels in Miami Beach, Florida—the Deauville Hotel.

Watching the multitude of the deaf guests who were dressed in the latest fashion—women in low-cut, clinging gowns with glittering jewelry and men in formal attire of varying colors, animatedly chatting in the expensively decorated and furnished hotel lobby, an officer of the Association remarked, "And they call this a deaf ghetto!"

The adult deaf community is the natural result of a people who seek their own kind for mutual pleasure and benefit, as witness the Chinatowns in the large cities, the Latin Quarters, the Bohemian sectors, the art colonies, the Nob Hill and Park Avenue colonies of the wealthy, the Haight-Ashbury hippie colony, and so on.

Although free and easy communication is the prime reason for the deaf adult's gravitation toward other deaf people, their other mutual problems and interests hold them together as well. They feel at ease with each other. Approximately 95 percent of deaf adults marry deaf partners.

Although it may be said that communicative barriers are holding the deaf together and away from the outside world of the hearing, these barriers are far from inviolate. Most of the deaf have warm friends among the hearing—from familial contacts, acquaintances made at the job, and so forth. They enjoy some social activities with their hearing friends. However, very few of these deaf adults really find it possible and enjoyable to integrate with their hearing friends and devote all their social life to them. No normal, self-respecting deaf adult likes to find his rapport with his hearing friends repeatedly cut off when they turn to their other hearing friends and resume their ordinary conversation, which the deaf persons usually finds to be very difficult and upsetting to follow.

It has been found that a rough yardstick of the deaf population in any given general population would be slightly more than one-tenth of one percent. Therefore, if a metropolitan area boasts a population of four million, we can be pretty sure that there are a little more than 4,000 deaf people residing there. Of course, in some areas there may be other factors serving to make the deaf population larger or smaller than the average. For example, the deaf population of the Washington metropolitan area is dominated by the oldest post-secondary institution for the deaf—Gallaudet College. The high caliber of its deaf staff members and students has served to attract many deaf adults to the area in the anticipation of a rewarding social life. Moreover, many of the Gallaudet College graduates have preferred to settle down nearby in order to maintain their contacts with their Gallaudet friends. Therefore, the Washington deaf population is much larger than the average.

No matter how large a deaf population may be in any given area, it is still only a very small fraction of the general population, and therefore maintains the warm, close-knit, and folksy atmosphere of a small town or village where everyone is acquainted with everybody else. Anything that deaf individuals do is of interest to all the others, and the more well-known they are, the greater the interest! Although this means that deaf persons cannot be too indiscreet, at the same time they have the warm and cozy feeling that when they die, their funeral processions will be longer than the average.

The very nature of the closely-knit deaf community usually spawns many opportunities for social activities. There is a wide range of them for the deaf adult to choose from: local chapters of national or state organizations of and for the deaf, local social clubs with their own halls, religious groups, athletic teams and leagues, recreational groups, private group meetings at the members' homes in rotation, and private social gatherings. Between these social events, the average deaf adult usually has most of his weekends filled up, not to say anything of week nights!

Although the adaptation of teletypewriters for use on home telephone lines has been a big boon, the telephone is not the convenient and dependable instrument with the deaf that it is with the hearing. Therefore, the deaf spend more time driving around to pay social calls on their friends and to do necessary personal errands. In view of the above, it is not surprising that the average deaf family home usually shows much more activity than their hearing neighbors; there are more visiting automobiles in front of their house than any other home in the neighborhood, and they are more frequently invited out than their hearing neighbors.

The average deaf community is so closely-knit that it is usually very difficult for deaf persons to draw the line when they wish to plan for a private occasion. Whenever a deaf couple is given a housewarming party at their new home, a crowd of 100 or more is not uncommon. A deaf twosome are very lucky if they can limit the attendance at their wedding to 150 or 200. Prospective hosts often hesitate for a long time before throwing open their house for a New Year's Eve party, for it is quite impossible to limit this lively event to fewer than 50, 75, or even 100 persons.

In nearly every large city there is at least one club for the deaf. Although some of these clubs own their premises, most of them rent halls. Some pay monthly rent for the full use of their quarters, but the others meet only once or twice a month. These organizations usually have a difficult time meeting their expenses, for their deaf members on the average cannot afford to pay dues large enough to take care of all the desired expenditures. In addition, the "gimme" attitude of many of them has not accustomed them to taking up their fair share of the burden if it means making some personal sacrifices. Therefore, except for a few which are endowed, these clubs usually have to be content with inadequate facilities in undesirable neighborhoods. Since the only qualification for membership in these clubs is deafness, all kinds of people congregate there. This tends to discourage some types of deaf people from patronizing the clubs, for they know that they are sure to find some undesirable characters there.

The various religious denominations have not neglected the deaf. Their services to the deaf range from providing an interpreter for a few deaf parishioners at Sabbath services once a month to having a separate church with a full-time minister for deaf members. Certain denominations go farther than others in recruiting and training deaf pastors for their deaf members. In many instances the deaf are too few to warrant full-time services, so the church will arrange for a part-time minister or lay reader. The Lutheran Church pioneered the development of a very successful senior citizen housing for the deaf in Los Angeles. The Pilgrim Tower, consisting of over 100 units, has a long list of prospective deaf tenants waiting for a vacancy. The Catholic and Lutheran Churches are taking the lead in providing parochial schooling for deaf youngsters. In certain areas of the country, the Jewish deaf are very active. They not only have their own synagogues, but also social halls. In New York City, they have a senior citizen housing unit named the Tanya Towers.

The deaf belong to countless athletic organizations and groups in which they can compete not only with other deaf teams but also with hearing groups.

There are also numerous opportunities to indulge in civic activities because a close watch has to be kept for possible violations of the civil rights of the deaf, and the social structure of the deaf is bottom heavy with indigent or near-indigent persons needing help in obtaining available welfare and other services.

It goes without saying that the present status of the deaf leaves much to be desired; it will be a long struggle before the deaf can hope to achieve first-class citizenship.

Organizational Patterns

Dr. Boyce Williams, Director, Deafness and Communicative Disorders Office, Rehabilitation Services Administration, aptly described the changing pattern of the organizations of deaf adults in the *Guest Lecturer Series* at the North Carolina School for the Deaf as follows:

> It is convenient and understandable to weigh the social structure of today in terms of organizations. We have seen the deaf community grow organizationally . . . to an impressively larger network. However, the most significant growth is found in the action programs of the various organizations.
>
> The main thrust of each national organization has been quite restricted in scope and depth. Most activity revolved around the planning and conduction of periodic business-social conventions. Between conventions, committees carried on assorted duties after a fashion. Although considerable energy was expended and good thinking demonstrated in all of this work, it had the usual characteristics of much voluntary effort, noble in intent but woefully short in performance.
>
> Under the leadership of deaf professional persons, a number of these organizations have responded magnificently to unfolding opportunities that stem from public program needs by elevating their organizations to the level of the vendor of the services sought by public agencies. . . . Another basic advance lies in the establishment of a continuing central office for one large organization in its own building with full-time staff.
>
> Government, in providing partial support for these fundamental moves, is not only amply rewarded by the extent and quality of the services it receives, but is simultaneously increasing its ability to accomplish its mandate. This increase is in direct ratio to the extent that these activities have eliminated ignorance, apathy, and ineffectiveness in the deaf community in favor of awareness, interest, participation and demand.
>
> The specific actions that organizations of deaf people have undertaken and carried out have grown in frequency as the abilities of deaf leadership have been demonstrated successfully. It

should be said at this point that these abilities have always been there. The only new base to this vital advance is the creation of opportunities for deaf people to assume leadership roles as government and program administrators have awakened to the superior manpower deaf leaders provide.

It would be very difficult, if not impossible, to mention every organization run by deaf adults in the United States. Probably the best source of this information would be the annual directory of programs and services published annually by *American Annuals of the Deaf*. However, I would like to include here brief resumes of several organizations of deaf adults which are national in scope, mention their affiliates, and describe a few groups which are distinctive in their make-up or objectives.

Probably the oldest national organization is the National Association of the Deaf (NAD). It was organized in Cincinnati in 1880, and continued as a "bedroom" organization until 1950 when Dr. Byron B. Burnes, who was the president then, made arrangements for office space with a public relations agency in Chicago, Illinois. This was so successful that a move to Berkeley, California, was necessary. There the president could supervise the operations of the first full-time office and its manager. It soon grew into four rooms and took on an additional office worker. In 1964, the home office was moved to Washington, D.C., and the first full-time Executive Director appointed to manage the operations.

The NAD now has 47 state associations affiliated with the Association and a membership of approximately 18,000. It has actively concerned itself with various problems, such as discrimination against deaf drivers, excessive rates of liability insurance for deaf drivers, educational practices, obtaining equal vocational opportunities for the deaf, and other matters. The NAD is also involved with the problems of deaf people around the world through affiliation with the World Federation of the Deaf.

The NAD directed the first census of the deaf in 40 years for the United States Government. The results were published in

1974, and the information has proved to be extremely valuable. It formed a research arm, Deaf Community Analysts, Inc., which has conducted surveys, evaluations, projections, market research and product evaluation, and workshops. An Education Section is being formed. It is to be hoped that this group will play an important part in influencing future educational policies as the deaf consumer should be in the best position to know what comprise effective educational practices.

The Association provides the sole support for a Legal Defense Fund which is having a great impact. Some recent examples include guaranteeing the right of deaf prisoners to interpreting services, establishing the rights of deaf persons to interpreting services in offices of state service bureaus, forcing a state welfare department to install a TDD to accommodate foster parents who are deaf, providing assistance and advice to parents throughout the nation in cases involving rights under Section 504, P.L. 94-142, and other similar laws. One of the most important actions of the Fund was to win a decision in a U.S. Court of Appeals which establishes the fact that institutions of higher learning are obligated under Section 504 to provide interpreter services to deaf students.

In order to combat the general "gimme" attitude of deaf students in various educational programs and to build into them an awareness of their responsibilities as deaf adults and citizens of the world, the National Association of the Deaf started a Junior NAD movement by establishing chapters in various schools for the deaf. This has grown to the present 94 chapters and a membership of 3,200. It sponsors annual Youth Leadership camp sessions at Swan Lake Lodge, Penguilly, Minnesota. It sponsors biennial national conventions and annual regional conferences.

The National Association of the Deaf sponsors the Communication Skills Program, which has been responsible for initiating classes in American Sign Language, publishing

instructional books, conducting workshops to explore the
linguistic aspects of sign language, etc. The Program is also
coordinating a five-year project, the National Consortium of
Programs for the Training of Sign Language Instructors. Sign
Instructors' Guidance Network (SIGN) started in 1975 as the
first effort in improving the quality of sign language teachers,
shown by evaluation and certification. The National Symposiums on Sign Language Research and Teaching are gaining
popularity with each successive convention. The third one was
held in Boston in October, 1980. (See comments on linguistics
in Chapter 10.)

As a measure of the National Association of the Deaf's growing effectiveness and influence as the prime organization of
deaf consumers, a branch office has been established in In-
dianapolis, Indiana, and other branches are in planning stages.
The NAD held its centennial convention in Cincinnati, Ohio,
the site of its founding, in 1980. A record-breaking crowd of
deaf citizens as well as a large number of hearing professionals
attended the gala event. A parade through downtown Cincinnati sparked a week crammed full of exciting shows, pageants,
workshops, and exhibits, as well as business sessions. Several
other organizations by and for the deaf joined the once-in-a-
lifetime occasion by holding their own conventions either con-
currently or immediately afterwards.

American Deafness and Rehabilitation Association, formerly the Professional Rehabilitation Workers with the Adult
Deaf, is a group of professional workers with the deaf in
various categories who are making use of this avenue to report
on their own activities and to exchange information and ideas.
Their present activities include the publishing of the quarterly
Journal of Rehabilitation of the Deaf and a monthly newsletter, the
holding of biennial conferences, special workshops and
professional-interest sections, and serving as a resource for information on professional aspects of deafness. Their future
plans include certification of counselors for the deaf and

facilities in the area of deafness. This group has a membership of approximately 700.

Another group which is achieving a vigorous growth and which is playing a vital part in updating educational philosophy and processes is the International Association of Parents of the Deaf (IAPD). It has a home office, with an executive director, in the Halex House, the home of the NAD. IAPD supports the total communication concept for deaf children and works closely with the NAD, the foremost group representing deaf adult consumers. The IAPD sponsors a publication titled *The Endeavor*.

The next oldest national organization is the National Fraternal Society of the Deaf (NFSD), which antedated the NAD in the establishment of a full-time office and staff. NFSD was established because of discrimination against deaf citizens in the issue of insurance policies during the last part of the nineteenth century. Now it has nearly 14,000 members in 120 divisions in 37 states and Canada. The total insurance in force exceeds $23 million, and is backed by assets of $6.5 million. The business is administered from a large and modern office building in Mount Prospect, Illinois, by a full-time staff of 11 persons. The administrators, who have full policy-making powers, are all deaf. The NFSD has its own Hall of Fame to reward members for service in their divisions and community. It also gives 10 annual scholarships to members entering postgraduate study, annually awards a $50 U.S. Savings Bond to a graduate in each school for the deaf, and publishes a bimonthly magazine, *The Frat*.

The Gallaudet College Alumni Association (GCAA) was founded in 1889, and is composed of the alumni and former students of Gallaudet College, the only accredited liberal arts college for the deaf in the world. It has about 2,500 life members and is indirectly one of the most influential organizations of the deaf because its members have taken up leadership roles in almost every other organization of the deaf. The GCAA has 48 chapters all over the U.S. and Canada. It is presently in a fund drive to restore and renovate Gallaudet's nineteenth century gymnasium into an Alumni House.

The American Athletic Association of the Deaf (AAAD) was founded in 1945 and has seven regional affiliates and about 160 local member clubs of the deaf all over the country. It conducts annual regional and national tournaments in basketball and slow pitch softball, and biennial volleyball tournaments for men and women. In the plans are national golf tournaments. The AAAD also sponsors the U.S.A. team in the quadrennial World Games of the Deaf. These games are similar to the Olympic Games except that all participants are deaf. There are also regional organizations relating to particular sports, such as bowling, softball, skiing, and golf.

There are national religious groups serving deaf citizens. Probably the largest is the International Catholic Deaf Association, which is affiliated with the Roman Catholic Church. There are local chapters, and many priests and lay workers are trained to communicate with deaf Catholics. The National Congress of Jewish Deaf was organized in 1956 and has held biennial conventions ever since. It has 11 affiliate groups serving about 3,000 individual members. The Episcopal Church, American Lutheran Church, Lutheran Church-Missouri Synod, Assembly of God, as well as Baptists, Methodists, Mormons, and other denominations have their own groups for the deaf. The Roman Catholic and Lutheran Churches each conducts several schools for the deaf as well. The Episcopolians and Baptists permit deaf men to be ordained as ministers. However, the first deaf Catholic priest in American was recently ordained, and to my knowledge at least one deaf man became a rabbi. Unfortunately, his untimely death left the rabbinate devoid of deaf persons.

The Michigan Association of the Deaf was probably the first state organization of the deaf to establish its own full-time office. Since then several other state groups have followed suit with their own home offices.

In the last few years special social service agencies offering comprehensive services to deaf citizens have mushroomed all over the country because the long-time needs of the deaf community for social assistance have only recently been discovered and recognized by governments—federal, state, and local. This is especially gratifying because the deaf have long been ignored and left without assistance by public social service agencies although they have borne their share of the taxes which have supported these agencies. With a few exceptions, these special agencies started out as small self-supporting operations by the adult deaf community.

Although governmental assistance has made it possible to establish some of the homes and housing facilities for deaf senior citizens in the country, the other establishments were started and are still maintained by the deaf community itself. Perhaps the showpiece is the Columbus Colony, Inc. (Ohio) which was made possible by a housing grant from the federal government. In the colony are 106 rent subsidized apartments, a 100-bed skilled nursing home, and 10 family cottages. Projected are a chapel, an activity center, a crisis center, opportunity houses for various purposes, a research center, and a clinic.

10 The Economic Aspects of Deafness

The Employment Situation

It is impossible to mention in a single chapter all the factors which are responsible for the current economic status of deaf adults. Therefore, several generalizations will have to suffice. There is a wealth of resource material on this topic, for the dumping of young deaf adults on the labor market by their educational programs has created many unusual problems not only for the deaf persons themselves but also for concerned professionals such as social workers, vocational rehabilitation counselors, job placement officers, and welfare workers.

If I should be compelled to limit my description of the current economic status of deaf adults to a single word, the word I would choose would be *"underemployment."* The lamentable thing about this is that underemployment is *not* an inevitable result of deafness; the handicap itself is the least of possible causes. There is no reason why a deaf person cannot perform the duties of any position to the full satisfaction of his supervisor except when the duties require frequent telephone communication and/or oral conversation, such as those of a telephone operator or an interviewer (with hearing people). There are a growing number of instances where the qualifications of prospective deaf executives or administrators for certain positions are such that it would be a sound business practice to hire secretaries who can double as their interpreters. In some instances even hiring full-time interpreters would be the best and most productive action to take.

To return to the current economic status of deaf adults—that of underemployment—while investigating possible causes for it, I came up with the following chief reasons:

1. Inadequate education
2. Inadequate social adjustment

3. A poor public image
4. Poor service by programs that should serve the adult deaf
5. Isolation of deaf adults

These are the inevitable results when communication among deaf children is restricted by hearing educators, and when the educators set themselves up as the spokespersons for the general deaf community even when they rarely bother to maintain contacts with deaf adults.

These problems were bad enough during the heyday of the industrial age, when there were many opportunities for workers with limited educational backgrounds to take over positions on assembly lines or at automatic machines which turned out identical parts at a furious pace, but these difficulties are becoming graver for deaf adults now that the age of technology is fast advancing upon us.

The Babbidge Report has this to say about the problem:

> . . . This is not to suggest that the quality of vocational programs has deteriorated, but rather that the increasing complexity of our world of work has left the field of vocational education lagging, and not alone in the programs for the deaf.
>
> Requirements that formerly could be met by secondary or even elementary school offerings are decreasing. Vocational training and education requirements that require post-secondary school offerings are increasing. (p. 19)

Table A from Vernon's article in *Rehabilitation Literature,* pp. 258-267, gives a good picture of the vocational status of deaf adults. The grim story that this table presents is due not so much to the handicap of deafness as it is to the downgrading, undereducation, and undertraining that deaf children and youth have been getting in their programs.

Unless something drastic is done to change the prevailing educational practices, the employment picture for deaf people will worsen. In Mindel and Vernon's book, a labor authority is quoted to the effect that within ten years unemployment among deaf workers will be about 70 percent, and most of the

Table A. Comparison of the Vocational Status of Deaf and Hearing Persons

Vocational Status	Deaf	Hearing
Manual labor	About 87 percent	Less than half
Manufacturing	Over half, most in manual labor	About one-fourth of whom (25 percent) are at management level
White Collar (Professional-Technical)	17 percent Crammatte states this to be an over-estimate	Over half
Urban Workers	Unknown	70 percent
Unemployed		
1. Washington, D.C.		
White men	4.3 percent	3.1 percent
White women	7.4 percent	1.9 percent
Negro men	16.9 percent	5.6 percent
Negro women	41.2 percent	5.7 percent
2. Southwest U.S. Young deaf adults	25 percent	11.2 percent
3. New England Young deaf adults	17 percent	11.2 percent
Civil Service	Exact data not available but percent is small	15 percent

remaining 30 percent will be "dead-ended" in various unskilled and menial jobs.

In their book *They Grow in Silence,* Mindel and Vernon mention some major trends which are the most likely to contribute
toward the somber future for deaf workers. They follow:

1. There has been a shift from manual, semiskilled,
and unskilled jobs to many more white-collar jobs.

2. Of the 22,000 types of jobs listed in 1965, over
6,000 were new since 1959 and over 8,000 that existed
then are now extinct.

3. Educational requirements for employment are
rapidly increasing. The average worker today spends 33
percent more years in school than his predecessor, and
this trend is increasing.

4. Employment in the service sector will experience
the fastest growth. (pp. 102-105)

Perhaps indicative of the present efforts to upgrade opportunities for future deaf workers is the present rapid growth of
post-secondary programs serving deaf youngsters from a few to
many locations all over the country. Despite these worthy efforts to cure the ills of underachievement, preventive measures
would be much more effective; therefore, the traditional emphasis on the development of speech and speechreading in the
primary and elementary grades and the downgrading if not
outright exclusion of other academic skills should be modified,
and essential skills, such as mathematics, language, and allied
subjects, pursued more vigorously. This, of course, means the
employment of more facile means of communication with deaf
children than that of the oral method alone.

Some Examples of the Handicapping Effects of Deafness on Employment Opportunities

Deaf youngsters might have obtained the best education and
training for their chosen vocations; they might possess the re-

quisite mentality for their jobs, and, due to an extensive public relations program, they might have found a minimum of discrimination by their current or prospective employers. However, in spite of the reduction or removal of these barriers to optimum employment opportunities, deaf persons still encounter further barriers because of public prejudice, which will take a very long time to overcome. I will give some instances of how deaf workers have been blocked from possible promotions or further benefits.

My deaf father was an example of what deaf entrepreneurs, no matter how insignificant their businesses might be, could face. He bought a small printing shop in San Francisco and tried to make it a profitable enterprise. However, running a highly competitive business proved to be a losing proposition for a man with a hearing loss, for his customers would come to him only if he could offer quality and price which were advantageous enough for them to contend with the inevitable difficulties in communication. Many of them did not even seem to consider this angle; my father was deaf, so he should be cheap. Period. Under those circumstances my father had to give up his shop and be satisfied with a steadily-paying job, with hearing bosses worrying about operation details.

I also know of a few businesses being run by deaf persons from a back room with hearing employees fronting for them. Unfortunately, these deaf proprietors have a very hard time finding hearing persons who have integrity to front for them. I have heard of hearing persons taking advantage of their deaf bosses by either taking over the control of the business, or misappropriating the funds. In some cases these deaf operators manage to skirt the problem by recruiting hearing members of their immediate families to front for them.

For 30-some years a close friend of mine has stayed on with a shop as a prized employee through several mergers until the business became a giant firm. A few years ago he achieved the position of being number one in seniority with that company.

During all those years many young men came into the firm and
were informally trained by my deaf friend, only to rise above
him to become his foreman, department head, and even shop
superintendent. And, still there is my friend, the same ordinary printer he was when he first joined the company, even
though he knows all that there is to know about the inside and
outside of his firm. Although he was sometimes asked to act in
the capacity of a temporary foreman, and he did an efficient
job, he never failed to find one or two hearing workers who
resented his authority.

The existence of deaf peddlers, or rather, beggar-peddlers,
who vend trifles such as needles, band-aids, or manual
alphabet cards for cash donations from a general hearing public
is mainly due to the frustrations and discrimination that they
have encountered in attempting to find employment. Most of
them have found it to be such a lucrative and effortless means
of earning a livelihood that they have abandoned any pretense
of seeking decent employment.

In addition to such examples as these, deaf workers face additional discrimination not only from their employers but also
from their coworkers and trade unions. Qualifying tests frequently rely heavily on verbal skills that average deaf workers
do not have. If deaf applicants do weather these obstacles to
their employment, they frequently become such productive
and valuable workers that their employers usually seek more
deaf employees. This will explain why some firms have such
concentrations of deaf workers while discriminatory practices
have kept deaf workers entirely out of some others.

Deaf Adults at Work
What can deaf workers do to earn a living? Many uninformed
persons have asked this question. The answer is: everything!
That is, when deaf adults are not required to communicate by
means for which they are not equipped or trained, as a part of
their job responsibilities, they are capable of any kind of work.

An excellent overview of possible tasks is the book, *The Deaf at Work,* published in 1967 by the California School for the Deaf at Berkeley.

Many of the projects for deaf adults supported by federal grants are directed by deaf persons. Most of the post-secondary programs for deaf students have deaf staff members, and many of them also have deaf administrators. Although state residential schools for the most part have long accepted deaf teachers, day schools or class programs have only lately started to accept deaf persons to administrative posts.

We can find deaf persons employed in professional fields as: research workers, psychologists, chemists, laboratory technicians, engineers, draftspersons, architects, librarians, computer programmers, mathematicians, social workers and various other career areas.

A list of trades in which deaf workers have achieved success is too comprehensive to detail here, but the following are some examples: electronic assemblers, machinists, lens grinders, carpenters, cabinet makers, bakers, printers, truck and bulldozer drivers, upholsterers, gardeners, body and fender men, typists, clerks, business machine operators, key punch operators, wig makers, post office clerks, sheet metal workers, warehousemen, fishermen, dry-cleaning operators, shoe repairmen, welders, and a thousand others.

Although deafness becomes a bigger handicap when one attempts to own and operate a business, there have been and are some successful ventures. Twin brothers who are deaf operated a very successful laboratory in Salt Lake City. A deaf man owned two expensive restaurants in a Detroit suburb in partnership with his hearing brother. There are several shoe repair shop owners, and I know of at least two dry-cleaning plants run by deaf adults. A deaf master baker owns and operates a bakery in California, with his children dealing with his customers. As far as I know, two deaf adults are in the advertising specialties business. Since farming is a business, we should also recognize many deaf farmers as successful business owners.

Talented deaf persons are also in fine arts—painters, sculptors, writers, and poets.

The long list of successful career people illustrates that with proper schooling, training, and public relations, deaf people can compete on a par with hearing workers.

The Economic Status

The economic status of deaf adults is directly connected with their employment situation. Therefore, except for a few cases, their economic distribution is considerably below that of the general population. Let me draw a picture of the general pattern of the living conditions of deaf citizens as I have seen them during the years of my participation in the deaf community.

Very few deaf persons may be considered to be wealthy. It is uncommon to find deaf families living in palatial homes, but when we do see these people, the first thought that comes to us would be that they are scions of wealthy families; that they inherited their present riches, for it is rarer than the proverbial hen's teeth to find deaf adults amassing wealth from ventures of their own making. Even if they have the talent and know-how, their deafness often works against any possibility of real success.

After the few wealthy deaf families, we have many well-to-do families whose householders hold well-paying jobs due to the fact that they are well-educated and highly trained. It is also possible that there are two pay checks in each household. They may live in custom-built houses, or in the more expensive tracts.

The great middle majority would be those who hold average jobs which enable them to live in lower middle class neighborhoods. In order to improve their own lot, many of these families include working wives and mothers who bring home a second pay check.

Although the unemployment situation among deaf adults is worse than that among hearing persons, I would say that current generous welfare practices would put unemployed adults on about the same par economically as those who perform the lowest-paid menial jobs. Therefore, I would feel safe in saying that the remainder of deaf adults, whether working in lowly jobs or unemployed, live in substandard housing, and are totally ignorant of gracious living. Their only pleasures may be going to the local clubs for the deaf to socialize, or to various events such as picnics, athletic contests and tournaments.

Dr. John E. Weinrich, Professor of Economics, University of Alaska at Anchorage, made some interesting observations about the economic costs of deafness. Through some complicated calculations, he found that the average hearing worker could expect to earn some $392,613 during his lifetime. Using the same figuring, he found that the average deaf employee could earn only $132,538 during his lifetime. Therefore, the cost of deafness is $260,075.

This steep price can and should be lightened by vigorous efforts to improve traditional educational and training programs so that they will become more meaningful and beneficial to deaf youngsters.

11 What Is Being Done for the Deaf

Each year the *American Annals of the Deaf* issues an updated directory of programs and services for the deaf. It is quite comprehensive, and lists thousands of programs now in existence for the benefit of deaf children and adults. I have no intention of repeating the list here, but I would like to mention, however, general trends of efforts to aid deaf adults, as contrasted with programs established by the deaf community itself and government-funded projects generated by those organizations which were mentioned in the chapter on the community of the deaf.

Postsecondary Educational Programs

Probably of interest to those concerned with deaf adults are postsecondary programs which have had recent and sudden growth. Currently, there are three programs offering full four-year collegiate work to deaf students.

Gallaudet College—Having celebrated its centennial in 1964, this is the oldest college for deaf students. It is located in Washington, D.C., scarcely a mile from the national capitol. It offers a general liberal arts program, including a preparatory year to make it possible for deaf students from secondary programs to go through a transitional period if they should not be ready to begin regular collegiate work. It also offers graduate programs for both hearing and deaf students who wish to work for master's degrees.

On the campus are also two exceptional programs which are subsidized by the federal government: the Model Secondary School for the Deaf and the Kendall Demonstration Elementary School. Both programs are mandated to try innovative methods in educating deaf children with the expectation that the nation's schools for the deaf will eventually profit by using the most successful features of these methods. These two programs are also available for practicum work to Gallaudet College students majoring in education and allied subjects.

National Technical Institute for the Deaf—Located on the campus of Rochester Institute of Technology (RIT) in Rochester, N.Y., NITD was established in 1968 and is totally federally funded, with a student population close to 1,000. It is filling a long-time need for a technical postsecondary program for deaf students. It offers training programs in technical fields such as art, printing, photography, business, computer science, and allied health and science careers. Multiple exit points are available options from certification to diploma and associate's degrees. Bachelor's and master's degrees can be earned by cross-registration into any of RIT's other nine colleges. Deaf students who qualify for these programs receive support services.

NTID has established a National Center on Employment of the Deaf which became operational in September, 1979. It serves as a national service agency and authority on the employment of deaf people in the U.S. It coordinates the development of national job opportunities in partnership with other postsecondary institutions, rehabilitation agencies, and employers and provides placement assistance to those organizations by establishing a job bank for deaf persons nationwide. The Center also provides information related to employing deaf persons, conducts active programs with employers on job analysis and job modification, and trains job placement professionals and employers who work with deaf persons.

California State University at Northridge—Formerly known as the San Fernando Valley State College, this institution started its work with deaf people with a Leadership Training Program for the Deaf, sponsored by a Rehabilitation Service Administration grant. Although this training program for administrative posts started with all hearing students, deaf applicants were later accepted.

This was probably the first educational or training program not only to involve the local adult deaf community in its practicum work but also to welcome participation by deaf adults in various workshops and meetings. The university later expanded its program to include four-year collegiate work, teacher training, interpreter training, summer Master of Arts work, and short-term projects. The University also initiated the Project D.A.W.N. and the Operation TRIPOD. The former carried on work in adult education through local deaf leadership, and the latter organized parents, deaf adults, and rehabilitation workers for effective action to improve existing programs for deaf children and adults.

In 1974, the National Leadership Training Program in the Area of the Deaf-Blind was started, but the funding ended after five years. The university was a pioneer in the training of interpreters, and is now providing intensive training in order to meet the growing demands for skilled interpreters. Another area in which the university also pioneered was utilizing telecommunications, and now it has a Telecommunications Training Center. In 1976, a new program designated as ''New Careers in Business'' was started to encourage deaf students to move into new academic or professional areas in which they have capability.

Community College Programs—Riverside City College was probably the pioneer in the development of community college programs for students who would have been unable to be successful at regular collegiate programs, but who still need and want further career training. A program was started there in the year 1961, and ever since deaf students from the State of California have attended the program. This concept was found to be valid, and other community college programs have sprung up, some with the aid of Social and Rehabilitation Service (now the Rehabilitation Services Administration) grants.

A recent release by NTID and Gallaudet lists all postsecondary education programs with their offerings.

Continuing Education

For years sporadic efforts have been made to institute adult education classes for deaf persons. The first serious effort was probably made in 1963 when the then San Fernando Valley State College made a concerted effort to start an area-wide adult education program by enlisting the assistance of its Leadership Training Program participants. At about the same time several adult classes were started in the San Francisco Bay region. As a result, adult education programs were started in other metropolitan areas, such as Washington, D.C.; Flint, Michigan; Kansas City, Missouri; and four communities in Wisconsin.

In order to push further efforts in adult education, the San Fernando Valley State College obtained a government grant for the D.A.W.N. project in which workshops were held for deaf leaders from all over the country to discuss ways and means of starting programs in their respective areas.

In the spring of 1972 Gallaudet College received funds to start a Continuing Education Center. A prototype adult education program was started in the greater Washington area, and has since been expanded to include forums with distinguished speakers and short-term programs on special-interest topics. This program seeks to open existing community adult education programs to deaf adults through the use of interpretive services. Through in-service training programs, disseminatin of materials, and sharing of planning and development costs, 7,000 deaf adults annually now benefit in programs from the San Francisco Bay area to Hartford, Connecticut, and from Milwaukee to Atlanta. In 1974, the Center opened its Office for Summer Programs and Extension. Among the most popular programs have been Family Learning Vacations. More than 486 families have participated in them.

Public Service Programs

In 1971 Gallaudet College established a Public Service office

". . . to respond to all requests for service assistance in a positive way, to recognize that Gallaudet College has an obligation to serve the nation beyond its students on campus, . . . to serve to the extent that funds, staff, and general resources permit."

This office sponsored a series of conferences either to solve problems or to improve and expand services, such as those of teletypewriter agents; of vocational and technical educators to develop new signs for technical instruction; of speech and hearing authorities to develop guidelines for deaf individuals who function orally in professional settings; of day class program supervisors to develop better utilization of specialized information, materials, and services; of professionals in the area of interpreting for the deaf to develop programs to supply trained interpreters to meet the needs of the deaf in the nation; and of a group of deaf community workers to develop increased utilization of regular services in behalf of deaf citizens.

Division of Public Services
In a reorganization recently, the Center for Continuing Education became the College for Continuing Education under the Division of Public Services. This Division also includes the following:

The National Academy of Gallaudet College offers training in deafness and other disabilities to professionals in such fields as medicine, law, architecture, engineering, and government. The Academy also administers the National Center for Law and the Deaf.

The Gallaudet College Press responds to the need for worthy publications of significant interest to persons associated with the field of deafness. Books and other materials include scholarly works, curriculum materials, works of a service nature, and artistic and literary works. The goal of the Press is to impact the broader deaf community through the dissemination of media, materials, and literature in such areas as rehabilitation, education, research, and vocational and social adjustment.

The Special School of the Future project, funded by the W.K. Kellogg Foundation, is designed to assist schools for the deaf in developing for themselves various roles as community education/regional resource centers on deafness to serve parents, deaf adults, public schools, and professionals in service agencies and training programs. Reception of the Kellogg grant of $1.4 million for the Special School program was one of the highlights in 1979. The five-year project will work with three different models of the special school for deaf students: The Atlanta Area School for the Deaf in Georgia (a day program), the California School for the Deaf at Fremont (a large residential program), and St. Mary's School for the Deaf in Buffalo, New York (a semi-private school).

Rehabilitation Services Administration
Elsewhere I have mentioned assistance rendered by the Rehabilitation Services Administration of the Department of Education through government grants. This vital agency has been largely responsible for the renaissance of deaf adults and their communities. Here are a few more noteworthy projects that the R.S.A. has sponsored, or is sponsoring.

Perhaps the oldest and largest project is the vocational rehabilitation of handicapped persons. This is a covering service for all handicapped persons, but in many locations there are special counselors for deaf clients, and special facilities in several other locations for them. This service includes diagnosis, treatment if necessary, special training if needed, occupational training, placement in a suitable job, and follow-up.

In order to implement these services to deaf clients the R.S.A. also sponsors training programs for vocational rehabilitation professionals at universities and colleges in Arizona, Tennessee, Oregon, New York City, Illinois, California, and the District of Columbia.

The agency is sponsoring many rehabilitation centers with important programs for deaf clients. A partial list of them follows: Boston, Brooklyn, Manhattan, Philadelphia,

Maryland, Virginia, West Virginia, South Carolina, Georgia, Alabama, Ohio (5), Indiana, Wisconsin, Arkansas, Iowa, Texas (2), Arizona, Los Angeles, San Francisco, Salt Lake City, Oregon, and Seattle.

There is a rapid growth of community centers for deaf adults to meet a long-time need. The R.S.A. is sponsoring facilities in Pittsburgh, Pennsylvania, and Seattle, Washington; but there are other which are locally sponsored in Wichita, Kansas; Detroit, Michigan; St. Louis, Missouri; Nashville, Tennessee; New York City; and possibly other locations.

The following description of the services being offered by the Pittsburgh Counseling Center in its brochure will give an excellent idea of the purpose of such centers:

> Clients are referred to community agencies available to the general population. These agencies are often not satisfactorily used by the deaf, either because the deaf are unaware of available services or because of a breakdown in service due to the problems of communication.
>
> Counseling at the Center covers a wide spectrum and includes: personal adjustment training, vocational, social, family, and marital counseling.
>
> Consultation services are rendered to community agencies, parents' groups, companies, schools, and private organizations who seek help in working with the deaf or families of the deaf.
>
> The Center provides interpreting for deaf persons needing this service in relations with employers, agencies, legal and governmental officials, and others. Interpreting services increase the effectiveness of community services available to the deaf.
>
> Deaf people often have inadequate knowledge about such things as Social Security, insurance, government benefits, educational requirements, training, etc. The Center provides a place where they can get proper assistance and information relative to their needs.
>
> The Center seeks to orient interested groups and agencies in understanding the nature of deafness, the rehabilitation of deaf persons, and related topics. This also includes free courses in the language of signs.

In the spring, adult education classes are held. The subjects offered are those directly related to the deaf population's education,
social, and economic interests.

The Rehabilitation Services Administration has also taken
part in an experimental project with the Wayne State University of Detroit, Michigan, in which deaf candidates were tested
for aptitude in legal work. Likely persons were urged to study
law and try for admittance to the bar. There are numerous
positions not requiring court appearances in that field which
can be filled by qualified deaf candidates.

The R.S.A. has worked closely with the National Institute
of Handicapped Research in preparing for a Research and
Training Center on Deafness. The agency is also helping the
NIHR to start a feasibility study for establishing a center for
producing and distributing to deaf individuals captioned video
cassettes in a broad range of educational, cultural, scientific,
and vocational programming.

Media Services and Captioned Films
In 1958 the Captioned Films for the Deaf program was
established by the Office of Education of the Department of
Health, Education, and Welfare. The original purpose was to
make available to deaf adults captioned Hollywood-type,
general interest films so that they could understand and appreciate feature motion pictures which other people have enjoyed for so long. As of July 1972, 1,255,000 deaf persons enjoyed 43,918 showings of 277 features. Later amendments
broadened the scope of the services to include educational
films, research in the use of educational and training films for
deaf children, and later extended these services to all other
areas of the handicapped. The establishment of a National
Center on Educational Media and Materials for the Handicapped was one of their projects. This program, now re-named
Media Services and Captioned Films, also included four
regional media centers for the deaf. Good examples of under-

takings designed to help deaf adults were a series of three films to improve communication between law enforcement officers and deaf persons, a special televised program on deafness, and a media-oriented program for occupational training.

Captioned Television

On Sunday, March 16, 1980, captioned television programs became a reality for the deaf citizens of the country. After years of technical research, dialogue, and negotiations, three national television networks, NBC, ABC, and PBS, started captioning a total of approximately twenty hours of prime time shows. (CBS is still working to develop its own system.) The biggest stumbling block to an earlier start to captioning programs for hearing impaired viewers was the commerical networks' reluctance to use open captioning because the other viewers objected to the distraction of seeing captions on their shows. It was only when a way was found to provide "closed captioning" (captions that do not show unless brought out by decoding devices) that deaf viewers could finally start to follow the dialogue and plots of the shows which they had been second guessing for so long, and hereby begin to enjoy them fully.

Sears is the only retail outlet who is selling decoders for approximately $250.00, and television sets with built-in decoders for around $500 to $600. A non-profit corporation, the National Captioning Institute, Inc., was established to select and caption programs. A location in the Washington, D.C., area, and another in the Los Angeles area are doing the work. Each area has its own advisory board, with several deaf members, to help with the selection of programs as well as to determine policies.

National Theatre of the Deaf

The seed of thought for a national repertory theater of the deaf had long lain dormant in the minds of deaf leaders, but it was not until 1965 that the National Association of the Deaf approached the National Foundation of the Arts and Humanities for a demonstration grant. Insufficient funds forced the Foundation to turn down the request. However, the next year the Vocational Rehabilitation Administrtion gave a $15,000 planning grant to the Eugene O'Neill Memorial Theater Foundation, Inc., of Waterford, Connecticut, to start a National Theatre of the Deaf. David Hays was selected to be the project director.

The project thrived under the astute management of Hays; summer courses in theater were started and road tours planned. Early in 1967 the Federal government gave a $331,000 three-year operating grant to the Theatre. The purpose was not only to expose the public to the acting abilities of the deaf but also to demonstrate that deaf workers can be employed in theatrical occupations, such as set design.

Since then, the National Theatre of the Deaf has made not only a national reputation for itself, but also won worldwide renown through trips abroad.

Though the Theatre has won wide acclaim for its presentations, such as "Kasane," "Gianni Schicchi," and "The Critic," it really came into its own when it presented an originally-executed presentation, "My Third Eye," which portrayed the various problems of deafness and the hearing public's reaction to that handicap.

The Little Theatre of the Deaf is an off-shoot project, using about five members of the troupe for presentations to children and youngsters.

Some positive effects of the appearance of the National Theatre of the Deaf on the scene include the employment of deaf actors, directors, and producers in successful productions, such as the well-known television show, "Sesame Street," the well-received television special, ". . . And Your Name Is Jonah," the Emmy winning series "End of the Rainbow," the

Broadway play "Children of a Lesser God," which won three Tonys, and many other landmark accomplishments in drama and media. Perhaps the most important effect of all is the improvement of the image of sign language and deafness, and the acceptance of signs by the general public as a legitimate and expressive communication modality.

Mental Health Services for the Deaf

A long-needed focus has been brought to bear upon the mental health problems of deaf persons, since restrictive practices in their education and development have caused more than an average number of mental and personality problems among deaf adults. Moreover, isolation and lack of communication have served to perpetuate the mental illnesses of deaf patients committed to facilities for the acutely ill. Government funds have made it possible to establish special mental health services for deaf persons at the Rockland State Hospital in New York, at the Langley Porter Clinic of the University of California Medical Center in San Francisco, at the St. Elizabeth's Hospital in Washington, D.C., and others.

However, probably the most exciting development in my estimation is the Community Mental Health Center for deaf persons at the Maimonides Hospital in Brooklyn, New York. For the first time I saw qualified deaf personnel perform group therapy sessions with low-verbal persons. The low-verbal deaf adults probably need professional help more than any other deaf group, but until that day I know of no qualified personnel who could communicate "on a gut level," and relate with these patients so that they could easily understand and cooperate.

Deafness Research and Training Center

The Deafness Research and Training Center was established in 1966 by a grant from the Social and Rehabilitation Service (now the Rehabilitation Services Administration) to New York

University. It is the only S.R.S.-sponsored research and training center exclusively concerned with deafness. The purpose of this center was stated in the grant as initiating research and training programs demonstrating "what can be done to allow the deaf individual proper evaluation of his potential ability to attain maximal skill in adapting himself to his environment and its changing characteristics, to find satisfaction in work and leisure activity, and to lead the fullest, most adequate life of which he is capable."

The Center has a formidable record of achievements to its credit. Among its research and demographic studies were the historic National Census of the Deaf, social and attitudinal aspects of deafness, television studies, career issues, and others. Its training program involved interpreters, counselors, psychologists, residential counselors, and rehabilitation workers.

The agency has also developed curriculum and materials for interpreting, sign language instruction and modification (for deaf-blind children), counseling, and some educational programs. Its advocacy efforts involved the needs of the aged deaf, continuing education, a model state plan for vocational rehabilitation, and others.

University of California Center on Deafness

The University of California Center on Deafness in San Francisco has been enabled to expand its services, mainly in the area of mental health, through funding from the Rehabilitation Services Administration, the California State Department of Health, the Department of Health, Education, and Welfare, and from private foundations.

The Center is presently engaged in four main tasks: direct mental health services to deaf people, their families, and agencies serving the deaf; research on deafness and mental health; advanced training in the mental health aspects of work with the deaf; and technical assistance to programs across the country requesting information and consultation in the area of deafness and mental health.

Professional Organizations in the Field of Education

Last but not least are organizations for educators of the deaf, which are probably the earliest-organized groups in the field of deafness. Since their inception, these groups have been dominated by hearing educators who gave short shrift to opinions, wishes, and needs expressed by deaf adults until comparatively recently.

The oldest and the most liberal group is the Convention of American Instructors of the Deaf (CAID) formed in 1850. This organization, which has a heavy representation from state residential schools, has been open-minded about methods of teaching since most residential schools practice "combined" methods of teaching. At present it has 4,200 members, a good proportion of whom are deaf.

The Conference of Educational Administrators Serving the Deaf, formerly the Conference of Executives of American Schools for the Deaf, which was founded in 1868, was apparently an offshoot of the CAID. This group meets annually—by itself every even-numbered year and jointly with the biennial conventions of American Instructors of the Deaf every odd-numbered year.

The CAID and the CEASD jointly sponsor the nation's oldest professional journal in the education of the deaf—*American Annals of the Deaf*. The *Annals* has been published continually since 1847. Its editorial policy has been liberal and up-to-date, reporting the latest trends in the education of the deaf.

The Alexander Graham Bell Association for the Deaf was organized in 1890 "to promote the teaching of speech, speechreading, and the use of residual hearing to deaf persons." Its philosophy has been strict oralism; the organization is dominated by hearing educators, mostly from day school or class programs. Participation was opened to deaf adults only recently with the establishment of the Oral Deaf Adults Section. Naturally, the prime requirement for membership in the Section is the practice of oralism as the main way of life. Any use of hands for formal communication is severly condemned by the Association, although some of its members have reluctantly admitted that the use of occasional "gestures" is sometimes necessary.

The policy of this organization is repugnant to me for I feel that the group is the epitome of the imposition of the values and will of the hearing majority upon a deaf minority. The comparatively few oral successes, about whom the *Volta Review* has printed glowing testimonials, do not make up for the many deaf victims who have fallen by the wayside. Nor is it noted that the few successes achieved are despite, not because of the system.

These three professional organizations have set up the Council on Education of the Deaf, composed of representatives from the organizations. Perhaps the most important project planned by the Council was the standards for the certification of teachers of the hearing impaired. Of the 18 professionals involved in the development of the standards, only three were deaf.

Unfortunately, the requirement for teachers of the deaf to develop communicative skills was watered down to mere recognition and understanding of various communicative modes including fingerspelling and the language of signs among seven or eight others. They are still not required to use communication which is highly visible and accurate to deaf children, even though this is the communication which is being used by at least 95 percent of deaf adults.

The requirements also fail to contain practicum experience which includes interacting with and getting to know deaf adults. If teachers of deaf children are unacquainted with typical deaf adults and the problems they are facing, how can they do a good job of preparing the children to live as deaf adults?

And so, deaf children continue to be short-changed because they will still have to contend with imperfect and elliptical communication and unrealistic teaching—except, of course, for those who are fortunate enough to be placed in total communication programs.

This failure of the Council on Education of the Deaf to be more realistic in its requirements may be due to the fact that the Council has not seen fit to invite the largest organization of deaf consumers, the National Association of the Deaf, to join the group and supplement the theories of educators of the deaf with feedback from the products of past educational programs.

Section 504

"Section 504" is a catchall phrase used to mean legislation enacted as a part of the Rehabilitation Act of 1973 by the Congress. This particular section provides that:

> No otherwise qualified handicapped individual in the United States . . . shall, solely by reason of his handicap, be excluded from participation in, be denied the benefits of, or be subjected to discrimination under any program or activity receiving Federal financial assistance.

Section 504 "thus represents the first civil rights law protecting the rights of handicapped persons and reflects a national commitment to end discrimination on the basis of handicap."

This law has started shock waves rippling throughout various industries, public facilities, government and private agencies, and other establishments. Incorporated in the law are provisions for access and reasonable accommodations to enable participation by handicapped persons. In the case of the deaf population, it means that telecommunication devices and use of interpreters are to be given serious consideration to enable these affected persons to enjoy equal employment opportunities or otherwise full participation.

Access to Telephone Services

Although for some time the deaf community has enjoyed the use of telecommunication devices (TDD), it was comparatively recently that the telephone industry has started to make special accommodations for deaf customers. Through legislation and action by public utility commissions, voluntary organizations, and the industry itself, these conveniences have become a reality:

(1) Special services for handicapped customers which are centralized in local offices.

(2) 24-hour repair service.

(3) Answering services which enable deaf customers to make voice calls.

(4) Special rates for long-distance calls to compensate for the much longer TDD calls.

(5) 24-hour operator assistance service which was started nationwide on June 29, 1980.

(6) Special TDD directories and special codes used in telephone directories to indicate TDD's.

(7) Free use of TDD's for deaf customers.

It is amazing to see how much and how quickly the public is responding to the needs of the deaf community, once they are alerted and motivated.

Linguistics of Sign Language

Perhaps the most exciting recent development is the increasing involvement of linguists in American sign language. W.C. Stokoe, Jr., was a pioneer in this aspect of research when he analyzed signs as simultaneous compositions of a limited set of handshapes, locations, and movements. In 1965 he published a dictionary of the language using novel symbols to identify each sign.

This sparked a widening of interest in the linguistic aspects of American Sign Language (ASL). Another important development was the establishment of a laboratory at the Salk Institute near San Diego, California, for systematic research of ASL. Papers and workshops emanating from this institute contributed to an increased understanding and subsequent respect for ASL as a *bona fide* language with its own inflections and syntax, rather than just a conglomeration of gestures, mime, and handshapes. This has helped us to realize that ASL is indeed the deaf person's native language which evolved from the particular features and needs of a culture, just like all the other languages of the world. A landmark publication in this field is *The Signs of Language* by Klima and Bellugi.

These discoveries have profound educational and psychological implications and bring out a strong rationale for the bilingual approach to educating deaf children. This development was responsible for the inception of the popular National Symposiums on Sign Language Research and Teaching.

I have tried to mention the most important efforts to advance the welfare of deaf persons which have been sparked by the government or people outside of the deaf community. There are many more programs which have not been mentioned here. The *Annals* Directory is probably the best source of information about these services.

12 My Life Story

It has been suggested that I write my autobiography in this book as the feeling was that it would help the reader to see the author in the context of this book. Before I proceed I would like to reiterate that my upbringing and environment do not resemble the usual milieu of a deaf child born of hearing parents who have had no previous acquaintance with deafness.

My story begins with the birth of my mother in San Francisco. Her parents were first cousins, and after a first child who could hear, they bore three deaf children in succession. They decided to stop bearing children but two more came about 10 years later and they had normal hearing. However, those two youngest offsprings died from childhood diseases. Therefore, I knew only one aunt who could hear. All three deaf children went to the California School for the Deaf in Berkeley. My grandmother and Aunt Julia learned sign language, so I was always very much a part of the family group every time we visited relatives.

My father, the oldest of four brothers, on the other hand, lost his hearing from spinal meninigitis. He had no deaf siblings, and we could not communicate with his family at all except one uncle who could barely fingerspell. Although he attended the same school my mother did, they did not become sweethearts until after they graduated. They were going together when San Francisco was hit by the big earthquake and fire in 1906. I remember being enthralled by stories about the experiences that they and their families met during that devastating time. They were married in my mother's home in 1908.

Although my brother Harry was born in San Francisco with normal hearing, a bout with whooping cough at age 18 months cost him his hearing. This was indirectly responsible for my parents' abandoning San Francisco for the more clement weather of the East Bay. I was born when they were living in Berkeley. However, my mother clung to her old doctor, who practiced in San Francisco. So, when she was to deliver, my mother went to San Francisco and I was born at the old Mt. Zion Hospital in that city. I was born deaf. When my parents discovered that both their children were deaf and would be going to the Berkeley school, they purchased a small house only seven blocks from the school campus. The proximity to home allowed both my brother and me to walk to school every day. However, the superintendent persuaded my parents to place me in the dormitory when I was a junior in high school, "so that I would become accustomed to being away from home." The adjustment would then be easier when I was ready to go to Gallaudet College in Washington, D.C., as anticipated.

It is evident from the above that I enjoyed a normal childhood free of any barriers or restrictions in communication. The Berkeley school was also an old and familiar place to me because my parents were there, too, and I was acquainted with not only the physical facilities but also many of the staff before I ever became a pupil.

An illustrious graduate of the school who later became a respected staff member was Theophilus Hope d'Estrella, the subject of a book now being written. He was a good friend of my parents' and became my brother's and my friend also when we entered school. A waif of Mexican ancestry, he was found on the San Francisco streets, and became one of the first pupils of the school when it opened in San Francisco in 1860. He remained on the school campus all his life, eventually teaching art and a special class of slow learning deaf children. He only left the campus to go to a nursing home to spend the last few weeks of his life. He came back to the campus for the last rites. The large chapel was jammed full of the many alumni of the school who remembered and revered him. He was a gentle man, much loved for his wise counsel as well as story-telling

hours during which countless youngsters enjoyed enchant-
ment. I remember enjoying conversations with the old man,
and going to his funeral when I was 11.

Another person of renown who was also a friend of my
parents was Douglas Tilden, also a graduate of the Berkeley
school who later gained fame as a sculptor whose works still
grace prominent locations in the San Francisco Bay Area, including the Donohue Mechanics Statue at Bush and Market
Streets. The Berkeley campus of the University of California
has Tilden's Football Player statue, and the school for the deaf
campus has a magnificent statue, named the Bear Hunt. I
recall being fascinated by the old maestro's mannerisms in
both actions and conversation. He knew that he was a genius
and subsequently displayed flashes of temperment which kept
his friends and admirers in awe and at a distance. Such was his
character even to the last day of his life in spite of the fact that
he was virtually destitute. So proud and dignified was he that I
never once saw him complain. A book about him was recently
published.

Such was my childhood. During those days there was extreme polarity between the "oralists" and those who enjoyed
manual communication. Therefore, my parents were particularly anxious that time should not be taken from my regular
academic work for oral training. Like many healthy deaf
youngsters I despised the hassles with the speech therapist, and
I was delighted to have my parents intercede in this. As a
result, I was ready to graduate at the age of 14 and went to
Gallaudet College in Washington, D.C., when I was barely 15.
I had a hard time adjusting to my new life due to my young
age. I did not really find myself until I reached my sophomore
year, which was the third year of Gallaudet's five-year
program.

I received my bachelor's degree when I was 19, in the middle
of the great Depression. I was offered a counselor's job at the
older boys' dormitory at my alma mater. I received my real

baptism of dormitory life then, starting with the supervision of about 100 of the older boys which included sending them to bed at specified times. Once you realize that during my first years many of those boys were older than I, you will understand that I had a rugged time. During those nine years I shared a daily 24-hour schedule with only two others, which meant that a weekly work load of 70 plus hours was common. Nevertheless, I enjoyed my work because it was stimulating to be partly responsible for the shaping of those boys' lives. I feel that those years were largely responsible for my later proficiency in handling discipline problems in the classroom.

After nine years, my superintendent assigned me to teach English in the high school department. Social studies and mathematics were added later, and eventually I specialized in mathematics.

Several years later I started a program for a master's degree in special education at San Francisco State University. In those days we never dreamed of demanding interpreting help with our classes. We had to be satisfied with gazing on the professor's countenance and trying to get along with the help of notes written by hearing classmates. Naturally, our chief source of information was the class texts and other reading assignments. An incident which occurred during those days may interest you. Occasionally we would be fortunate enough to have a hearing colleague from our school taking the same course. In that case, we would rely upon his generous nature to receive interpreting help in that class. This incident happened at a seminar on special education where a different guest lecturer appeared at each meeting to talk about a particular category of disability. One evening the wife of the professor in charge of the class came to speak about cerebral palsy. As usual, our colleague proceeded to interpret. However, after half an hour the lecturer spoke to him and he suddenly stopped interpreting. When we asked him why he stopped, he whispered to us that she had told him that his moving hands were extremely distracting and asked him to keep his hands quiet! During the break we went to her and explained why our friend was so busy with his hands. The poor woman became flustered and apologized to us. But, we continued to wonder how it happened that a specialist in the field should be so ignorant that she could not recognize sign language!

When there were four of us deaf students who were ready to graduate with master's degrees at the same time, it was so unusual that a San Francisco paper sent a photographer to take a shot of us marching together up to the platform to receive our degrees.

In 1954 I visited Gallaudet College at Christmas time, and met a young lady in her senior year. I was struck by her outgoing nature and her thoughtfulness for older visitors to the campus, which was unusual for youngsters her age. I found out that she had deaf parents which explained her outgoing nature. The geographical difference did not stop me from courting her long-distance. I took unto myself a wife two years after I met her. I had experienced life out of school for quite some time so I was pretty sure of my choice, but I have always wondered about her courage in marrying someone with whom she had had not much more than casual contacts during two years of long-distance courtship. However, I am quite sure that she never regretted her decision, and neither did I. Our happy union was blessed by the advent of two girls. Considering our heritage of deafness, we expected deafness in our children, and would have welcomed it, for it would have meant closer kinship in the family. As it was, the older girl, Sheila, was hearing. The younger, Lisa, was born with hearing, but contracted tonsillitis when she was a year old. The attacks repeated at monthly intervals until the doctor diagnosed that a family member must have been a carrier of the disease. After the three of us took antibiotics, Lisa became well, but showed a continuing loss of hearing.

In September 1970, when my children reached adolescence, my wife, Dot, obtained a teaching position in a special program for deaf children, and became the first deaf teacher in the

Oakland City Unified School District. It was apparent that her performance was more than favorable, for they hired another deaf teacher the next year. Dot taught for seven years before she became a victim of cancer. She died a year later in 1978.

In 1975 I was appointed to be the Coordinator of Continuing and Community Education in the San Francisco Bay Area. My work was totally different from teaching and quite stimulating. I traveled all over the bay area, participating in various community activities. I started an annual observance of "Deaf Awareness Month" each May. I feel that awareness efforts have been very productive because of their long-term effects. In the summer of 1979, with both children away in college, and having completed 41 years of service at my school, I decided to retire.

This is the story of my life so far. Strangely enough, I am finding that my days are full for the most part, although on occasion I have felt some loneliness and unrest. It has not been easy to reconcile myself to a life devoid of the companionship and care that Dot had given to me.

13 In Retrospect

This has been a chronicle of deafness as seen through the eyes of a deaf adult who has known neither the conveniences nor joys of normal hearing or speech. However, the wheel of fortune descried that I should be born of a deaf family; therefore, I never noticed my own handicap nor came up against discriminative or unfair treatment until I began my own personal contacts with hearing people when I entered school.

With this as my background, it was to be expected that I felt more handicapped from the treatment I received at the hands of hearing people than from my deafness. During all the years since this initial impression, I have become more firmly convinced that the real ills of deaf people lie more with minority group dynamics than with their deafness, and that these problems will not cease until the attitude toward deafness by the hearing majority changes.

During the last decade it has begun to happen; the hearing public has begun to be aware that their traditional treatment of deafness has not produced the results they had anticipated. During the same period of time, several other minority groups became more vocal and militant, and good things began to happen to them. And, as responsible deaf leaders became more articulate, hearing political and community leaders listened to them. Good things began to happen to deaf citizens, too.

The government has begun to be more aware of the principles of consumerism, so more and more deaf persons have been asked to serve on advisory committees and/or in positions where they could participate in decision- and policy-making, for no one knows more about a particular problem than one who is directly affected by the problem. Though it was a relatively unknown practice until recently, several deaf persons have been appointed to chief executive positions in educational programs for deaf children.

A deaf educator coined the term "total communication" for a new concept in educating young deaf children. Success begat success and total communication is sweeping the nation like wildfire. Many homes where young deaf children are living are using total communication, and these children are enjoying total involvement with their families, a situation very rarely experienced before by deaf children having hearing parents. This total involvement is carried over into educational programs employing total communication, and their parents and teachers could see that the children are different and more nearly normal in their progress and achievement.

New projects utilizing novel concepts are infiltrating the adult deaf community. Special television broadcasts for deaf citizens are increasing in number and quality; the shows put on by the National Theatre of the Deaf, which are intended for the edification of the hearing public, are also enjoyed by deaf audiences; and cultural opportunities are increasing for deaf adults through local efforts by continuing education agencies. The growing number, availability, and professionalism of interpreters for the deaf mean that many programs which formerly limited their appeal to hearing audiences are now "open sesame" to deaf audiences.

Long a small minority in the ranks of traditional educators, our hearing friends who obtained their empathy for deafness from close contacts with deaf people, such as being members of families with deafness, or because of a rare knack for understanding, find their numbers now being swelled with newcomers to the field who, along with their training, have had practicum experiences not only with deaf children but also with local adult deaf communities. And, deaf adults are finding many more new hearing friends and champions.*

---

*Many hearing readers of this book have asked the same question over and over again, in different forms. An over-all version would resemble this:

As long as this trend continues, I cannot see anything but a brighter future for our deaf children and future adults if we continue our vigilance against opposing forces who wish to maintain the *status quo* for selfish reasons. As long as our deaf children continue to enjoy the freedom and relaxation of the total communication philosophy, I am confident that they will not only read, write, and figure better, but also speak and read lips better. And, these children will grow up to be our future deaf adults.

"You have shown anger at the treatment of the deaf minority by the hearing majority, and criticized the actions of hearing professionals working with deaf people. Now, what would you suggest for me, as a hearing person, to do if I wish to mingle or work with deaf persons?"

It would be impossible for me to give a definite answer to this question, with a suggested sequence of steps to take, 1, 2, 3, etc. I believe that, in the final analysis, it is a matter of having the right attitude toward deaf persons. If you treat this venture as an ego trip, with missionary zeal, or as an easy career opportunity, it would be wiser for you to forget working with the deaf, and look elsewhere to satisfy your need for self-satisfaction. We can get along very well without hearing persons who "do good," patronize us, or use us.

However, if you do have a real desire to know the deaf as real persons, and to regard them as equal individuals whose physical restraints have obliged them to communicate not only in a different language but also a unique modality, and subsequently develop their own culture, and if you are also willing to be totally immersed in that language and culture, then I am quite sure that you will be welcomed by the deaf community.

At the same time, there would be a limit to this involvement; from past experience, we are usually wary about going all the way toward including a hearing newcomer in our community. The question we first ask ourselves is: "What is he getting out of this?" Once we are convinced that he is genuinely interested in becoming our friend, we usually welcome him with open arms. At the same time, naturally, we do not expect him to foresake his own society.

Glossary

Note: Some of the terms used in this manuscript may be subject to different interpretations. Therefore, these terms are listed below with the denotations which were used for them.

Ameslan—An abbreviated form of the phrase, American Sign Language, the traditional manual communication used by deaf people. This communication has its own syntax. Fingerspelling is used whenever necessary.

Communication—A transmitting; a giving, or giving and receiving, of information, signals, or messages by speech, gestures, writing, etc.

Deafness (Deaf)—A condition in which the residual hearing, if any, is not usable; perceivable sounds have no meaning to the individual.

Fingerspelling—A method of communicating in which the hand or hands are used to show the 26 letters of the alphabet. Thus, exact words and sentences can be spelled out with the hand.

Full communication—An open, facile communication where meaningful responses are the rule, not mere monosyllabic utterances, such as "Yes," "No," "Mommy," etc.

Hard of Hearing—Hearing-impaired persons who are able to utilize their residual hearing through amplification to such a degree that they are able to carry on normal oral communication with a minimum of difficulty.

Hearing Impairment (Hearing Impaired)—These terms are meant to include every person who has a hearing problem, whether hard of hearing or deaf.

Lipreading—Implies a concentration on lip movements only.

Manual—Using sign language and fingerspelling, sometimes with the help of body movements and facial expressions.

Manual English—A system of communication in which both sign language and fingerspelling are used to follow the exact sequence, or syntax of the English language.

Oral—Communication efforts using speech and lipreading.

Oralism (Oral Method)—A situation in which communication is restricted to speech and lipreading, although writing and reading are also used. Sign language and fingerspelling are forbidden. Thus, the term, oralism, is differentiated from oral, which means merely the employment of speech and lipreading.

Residual Hearing—The amount of hearing a hearing-impaired person may have; it may be of some use or of no use at all. (See discussion on page 6.)

The Rochester Method of Communication—A method in which only oral communication and fingerspelling are permitted.

Sign Language—An ideographic system in which symbols are made with the hands to show entire concepts. Thus, if signs alone are used, it is difficult or impossible to follow the exact sequence of the English language.

Speechreading—Takes into consideration the context of the conversation, natural gestures used by a speaker, facial expressions, and other associational cues and lip movements.

Total Communication—A philosophy in which full communication is established through the employment of one or more methods, creating the most effective environment for the persons involved in the give-and-take of communication. Possible methods would be writing, reading, illustrating, amplification, speech, lipreading, sign language, fingerspelling, gestures, body movements, and/or facial expressions.

References

Adams, E.J., & Murphy, H.J. *Evaluation report of an experimental program for deaf and severely hard of hearing minors eighteen months to three years of age.* Report to the Office of the Los Angeles County Superintendent of Schools, 1971-72.

Albronda, M. *Douglas Tilden: Portrait of a deaf sculptor.* Silver Spring, Md.: T.J. Publishers, Inc., 1980.

Albronda, M. *Theophilus Hope d'Estrella.* Book in preparation.

Bangs, T. *Language and learning assessment.* Madison Communication Project, Santa Ana (California) Unified School District, 1968, 1969, 1970.

Best, H. *Deafness and the deaf in the United States.* New York: The Macmillan Co., 1943.

Brill, R.G. The superior I.Q.'s of deaf children of deaf parents. *The California Palms,* Riverside, Calif., School for the Deaf, 1969.

California Department of Education. *A proposed plan for the improvement of the education of the deaf and severely hard of hearing in California* (booklet).

Conant, J.D. *The comprehensive high school: A second report to interested citizens.* New York: McGraw-Hill Book Co., 1967.

Conference of Executives of American Schools for the Deaf. *Minutes of the 26th regular meeting,* 1954.

Conference of the Executives of American Schools for the Deaf. *Parent education* (brochure). Wisconsin School for the Deaf Press.

Crammatte, A.B. *Deaf persons in professional employment.* Springfield, Ill.: Charles C. Thomas, 1968.

Davis, H., & Silverman, S.R. (Eds.). *Hearing and deafness.* New York: Holt, Rinehart, & Winston, Inc., 1960.

Denton, D.M. A study in the educational achievement of deaf children. *Proceedings of the 42nd Meeting of the Convention of American Instructors of the Deaf,* 1965, 428-438.

Drake, H.D. The deaf teacher of the deaf. *American Annals of the Deaf,* March 1940, 150.

Fellendorf, G.W. Is oralism worth the effort? *The Volta Review,* September 1971, 352.

Gallaudet College. PL 94-142 and deaf children. A special issue of the *Gallaudet Alumni Newsletter,* June 15, 1977.

Gallaudet College. The 503 & 504 legislation. A special issue of the *Gallaudet Alumni Newsletter,* June 15, 1978.

Gallaudet College & National Technical Institute for the Deaf. *A guide to college/career programs for deaf students,* 1978.

Garret, J.F., & Levine, E.S. Communications difficulties of the deaf. *Psychological practices with the physically disabled.* New York: Columbia University Press, 1969.

Garrett, C., & Stovall, E.M. A parent's views on integration. *The Volta Review,* 1972, 338-344.

Garretson, M.D. *A question of relevance.* Paper presented at Region IV Conference for Coordinating Improved Rehabilitation and Educational Services for Deaf People, Knoxville, Tenn., 1969.

Garretson, M.D. The residential school. *The Deaf American,* April 1977, 19-22.

Goodman, M.J. *The deaf student in the hearing class.* Unpublished handbook for instructors, Golden West College, Huntington Beach, Calif., 1971.

Greenberg, J. *In this sign.* New York: Holt, Rinehart & Winston, 1970.

Hester, M.S. Manual Communication. *Proceedings of the Interior Congress on Educating of Deaf and the 41st Meeting of American Instructors of the Deaf,* 1963.

Hoerr, C.R. Try it—You'll like it. *The Volta Review,* 1972, 332-333.

Holcomb, R. Some "hazards" of deafness. *The Communicator,* Indiana School for the Deaf Parent-Teacher-Counselor Organization.

International Association of Parents of the Deaf, Inc. *Position papers.*

Jacobs, L.M. Of the confusion in the meaning of total communication. *The California News,* Berkeley, Calif., School for the Deaf, 1971.

Jensen, K.M., & Baldis, B.J. *Final evaluation: Experimental program for deaf and severely hard of hearing minors (18 months to 3 years of age).* Report to Fresno (California) City Unified School District.

Katz, Mrs. N. A parent's belief in using all avenues of communication. *The Deaf American,* 1967, 35.

Klima, E., & Bellugi, U. *The signs of language.* Cambridge, Mass.: Harvard University Press, 1979.

Kohl, H.R. *Language and education of the deaf.* Policy study 1, Center for Urban Education. New York: Center for Urban Education, 1966.

Levine, E.S. *The psychology of deafness.* New York: Columbia University Press, 1960.

Lowell, E.L. Research in speechreading: Some relationships to language development and implications for the classroom teachers. *Proceedings of the 39th Meeting of the Convention of American Instructors of the Deaf,* 1959, 68-73.

Lunde, A.S., & Bigman, S.K. *Occupational conditions among the deaf.* Washington: Gallaudet College, 1959.

McClure, W.J. Current problems and trends in the education of the deaf. *The Deaf American,* 1966, 8-14.

Meadow, K.P. Early manual communication in relation to the deaf child's intellectual, social, and communicative functioning. *American Annals of the Deaf,* 1968, *113,* 29-41.

Mindel, E.D., & Vernon, M. *They grow in silence.* Silver Spring, Md.: National Association of the Deaf, 1971.

Mitchell, S.H. *An examination of selected factors related to the economic status of the deaf population.* Unpublished doctoral dissertation, American University, Washington, D.C., 1971.

Montgomery, G.W. Relationship of oral skills to manual communication in profoundly deaf students. *American Annals of the Deaf,* 1966, *3,* 557-565.

Mow, S. How do you dance without music? *Answers,* James A. Little (Ed.), Santa Fe: New Mexico School for the Deaf, 1970.

Myklebust, H.R. *The psychology of deafness: Sensory deprivation, learning and adjustment* (2nd ed.). New York: Grune & Stratton, 1966.

National Technical Institute for the Deaf. New national center on employment of the deaf, *The Deaf American,* January 1979, 25.

Newman, L. See! see! see! see! *California Forum,* Teachers of Deaf and Hard of Hearing, 1968.

Newman, L. Teacher training. *The Deaf American,* 1969, *21,* 17-18.

Norris, A.G. (Ed.). *Deafness* (Vol. 2). Silver Spring, Md.: Professional Rehabilitation Workers with the Adult Deaf, Inc., 1972.

North Carolina School for the Deaf. Guest Lecturer Series, 1971.

Ottinger, P.J. Dr. David Denton: Total communication. *The Deaf American,* October 1971, 3-6.

Quigley, S.P. The influence of fingerspelling on the development of language, communication, and education achievement of children. *Proceedings of the 42nd Meeting of the Convention of American Instructors of the Deaf,* 1964.

Quigley, S.P., & Frisina, D. Institutionalized and psychoeducational development in deaf children. *Council for Exceptional Children Research Monograph,* Series A, 1961, *3.*

Rhodes, M.J. From a parent's point of view. *The Deaf American,* July-August 1967, 26.

Schein, J.D. *The deaf community.* Washington: Gallaudet College Press, 1968.

Schein, J.D., & Delk, M.T. *The deaf population of the United States.* Silver Spring, Md.: National Association of the Deaf, 1974.

Schlesinger, H.S., & Meadow, K.P. *Deafness and mental health: A development approach.* San Francisco: Langley Porter Neuropsychiatric Institute, California State Department of Mental Hygiene, and University of California, 1971.

Sharoff, R.L. Enforced restriction of communication, its implications for the emotional and intellectual devleopment of the deaf child. *The American Journal of Psychiatry,* 1959, *116.*

Stevenson, E.A. *A study of the educational achievement of deaf children of deaf parents.* Berkeley: California School for the Deaf, 1964.

Stokoe, W.C., Jr., Casterline, D., & Croneberg, C. *A dictionary of American sign language.* Washington: Gallaudet College Press, 1965.

Stuckless, E.R., & Birch, J.W. The influence of early manual communication on the linguistic development of deaf children. *American Annals of the Deaf,* 1966, *3,* 452-462.

United States Congress, Senate Committee on Labor and Public Welfare. *Hearings before the subcommittee on the handicapped.* 92nd Congress, 2nd Session, 1972, Part 2, H.R. 8395.

United States Department of Health, Education and Welfare. *Education of the deaf: A report to the secretary of health, education and welfare by his advisory committee on the education of the deaf,* 1965.

Vernon, M. The failure of the education of the deaf. *The Illinois Advance,* Jacksonville, Ill., School for the Deaf, 1968.

Vernon, M. Multiply handicapped deaf children: Medical, educational and psychological considerations. *Council of Exceptional Children Research Monograph,* 1968.

Vernon, M. Potential, achievement, and rehabilitation in the deaf population. *Rehabilitation Literature,* 1970, *31,* 258-267.

Vernon, M. *The role of the deaf teacher in the education of deaf children.* Paper presented at Gallaudet College, April 8, 1970.

Vernon, M., & Koh, S.D. Early manual communication and deaf children's achievement. *American Annals of the Deaf,* 1970, *115,* 527-536.

Vernon, M., & Makowsky, B. Deafness and minority group dynamics. *The Deaf American,* 1969, *21,* 3-6.

Wienrich, J.E. Direct economic costs of deafness in the United States. *American Annals of the Deaf,* August 1972, 446-454.

Appendix A

Seven Other Faces of Deafness:
A Panel Discussion by Deaf Adults

Seven Other Faces of Deafness*

Nowhere before has there been published the views of a rank and file group of deaf panelists expressing themselves openly and freely in sign language. Therefore, I was determined to organize such a panel discussion. In order to cope with this problem, I undertook the following procedure:

1. I selected the participants by using the following criteria: (a) they were products of schools or programs for the deaf who did not go on to college, with one exception who attended for only one year; (b) they represented divergent educational backgrounds.

2. I decided to solve the problem of recording the discussion by asking a deaf individual to record the statements of each panelist by writing them in freely translated English which should, however, show the same intent as the Ameslan used by the panelist. Therefore, I had seven recorders sitting across the table from the seven panelists. Each recorder thus had the time to give his full attention to his designated participant, and to translate quickly enough to keep up with the free exchange of ideas. In order to make the transcript as accurate as possible, I had the panelists check with their recorders after the discussion to see if their intent was shown intact in the written record. An interesting development occurred after I had chosen my recorders. I had based my selection on two criteria: (a) they should be able to read Ameslan well enough to get the intent easily, and (b) they should be able to write English well. It was not until the night of the meeting that we realized that six of the eight recorders had deaf parents.

---

*The genesis of the idea for this panel discussion, and also the title, was a seminar with deaf professionals which was held in Memphis, Tennessee, in 1972.

3. The meeting was set for Friday evening, April 10, 1973, and it was held in the Eagle's Nest conference room at the California School for the Deaf at Berkeley through the kind permission of the school authorities. I asked Mr. Jacob Arcanin, the Assistant Superintendent of the Berkeley school, to serve as an observer.

4. The names of the participants in the panel discussion follow, with their backgrounds given. The identity of each panelist's recorder is given at the end of each paragraph.

Mrs. Margaret Burroughs—Age 44. Born deaf. Attended Hawthorne and Hamilton oral schools in Oakland, California, leaving after ninth grade. Now working as a procurement clerk at the Presidio Army Base, San Francisco. Recorder: Miss Helen Arbuthnot.

Mrs. Jo Jacobs—Age 48. Lost hearing from whooping cough and measles at ten months of age. Hard of hearing. Graduated after ninth grade from the Alexander Graham Bell oral school in Cleveland, Ohio. Now working as a key punch operator at The Oakland Tribune. Recorder: Mrs. Lois Bullock.

Alfred Lowe—Age 67. Lost hearing at age five from measles. Hard of hearing. Attended an oral school at Aberdeen, Scotland, until graduation at age 14. A retiree now, his last job was as a stock clerk at the Rhodes department store in Oakland for 23 years. Recorder: Mrs. Judith Holmes.

Stephen McCullough—Age 27. Cause and age of deafness unknown. Attended oral schools, then the Kendall School in Washington, D.C., before coming to the Berkeley school where he was in the tenth grade. Presently a printer at the Sorg Company in San Francisco. Recorder: Harry M. Jacobs.

Enrique Marquez—Age 30. Began to lose his hearing after he fell from a horse at age eight. Became totally deaf at age 15. He was born in Mexico, and attended a missionary school for a short time. He could speak Spanish, but he could not write in either Spanish or English until he went to the Berkeley school at age 16. He graduated from the school at age 21, and is still the only literate member of his family. Recorder: Mrs. Patricia Zinkovich.

Lonnie May—Age 25. Cause and age of deafness unknown. Being a son of an Army man, he attended the Arkansas School for the Deaf first, then schools in Frankfurt, Germany, and Brighton, Sussex, England. He returned to the Arkansas School for a year, then attended the Berkeley school until his graduation. Dropped out of Gallaudet College after his preparatory year, and completed his freshman year at the Laney Community College, Oakland. Presently unemployed. Recorder: Mrs. Carola Rasmus.

Miss Sharon Negrini—Age 31. Lost hearing at age one from either a high fever or a fall. Attended the Louisiana, Georgia, and Texas Schools for the Deaf, dropping out of the latter after the sixth grade. Presently unemployed. Recorder: Mrs. Joyanne Burdett.

Mrs. Dorothy M. Jacobs functioned as the eighth recorder, keeping tab on the order of speakers.

Moderator: Let's go on with the discussion. As you know, I asked you to come here tonight so that you can contribute your feelings, opinions, and experiences pertaining to your deafness. Can you tell us what being deaf means to you?

Mr. Marquez: I do not want any pity; my only problem is communicating with the hearing. I am not perfectly happy, but contented enough with being deaf.

Mrs. Jacobs: I am not happy to be hard of hearing; I am always in between the deaf and the hearing. It is more of a problem being hard of hearing because hearing persons expect me to understand them. For instance, one time I happened to hear the phone ring despite the noisy machines around me. But, when I mentioned it to my supervisor, she began to think that I was lying about my hearing problem. I felt cheated because I could not explain my handicap so that my hearing co-workers would understand it. I would rather be deaf because I think it is less of a problem.

Mr. May: Since I was born deaf, I have never been sorry to be deaf except that I was curious at first about the appeal of music to hearing persons. I can feel the vibrations, and I see other deaf persons showing facial expressions when they feel music. I never had problems being deaf because as soon as I enrolled in school at five, my mother learned the language of signs. I have learned a lot by communicating with her.

Miss Negrini: I am rather disappointed that I did not receive enough education. I feel that I would have had more education if I were a hearing girl. I was very much spoiled by my mother, who pitied me because I was deaf. She thought I would not be happy at school, so she let me stay home most of the time. I would not return to school until Tuesday morning after a weekend at home, and I was permitted to stay home all week every once in a while.

Mr. Marquez: When I first went to the Berkeley school at age 16, I used hearing aids in both ears. I did not feel comfortable with them, and I was unable to understand speech with them. I became unhappy with them, so I quit wearing them. I was contented to be deaf, period. I talk with my parents in Spanish and they understand me. They do not speak English.

Mr. Lowe: Speaking of hearing aids, I had to wear one for the first time because the Rhodes Company ordered me to use one. I was never really happy with it, and I always took it off as soon as I got home.

Mrs. Burroughs: For a long time my mother did not want me to use sign language and forced me to wear a hearing aid. Three years ago I stopped wearing my hearing aid because it annoyed me to hear my shrill voice. Now that I am not wearing an aid, I think that I can talk better. And, I feel more comfortable and at peace not wearing a hearing aid.

Mr. McCullough: My parents were frustrated when they learned that I was deaf, and there was a lack of communication between us. I learned to use sign language at the Kendall School. My mother was against my using signs and when we moved to California, my father had to reach a compromise with my mother before she would let me enter the Berkeley school. My mother is now finally convinced that total communication is the best method, and strongly recommends that all deaf children be taught by this method.

Mrs. Jacobs: I still could not talk when I was five. Mother said that I got things I wanted by tugging at her skirt and pointing at them. I was put into a public school with a group of very slow learners. There were ten of us. I did not learn anything. A doctor tested my hearing and told my mother to send me to a school for the deaf. She wouldn't think of it. I still couldn't talk at seven. The doctor took me to the school for the deaf without my mother knowing it. When the school principal called her by phone, she was mad. She came to the school and found me crying because I was afraid of the doctor's stethoscope. The principal showed her around the school. Mother was not quite convinced and said she would put me back in the public school if I learned good speech. After two years I had picked up quite good speech, so she put me back in the public school. I cried because I didn't enjoy the hearing children. It was hard for me to understand them. I got lonely. They thought that I was a stubborn child, so back I went to the school for the deaf. I learned to communicate by gestures and home signs. I felt that a lot of education was lost because too much time was devoted to speech and lipreading. I graduated after the ninth grade, but I did not want to start high school at age 18 because I would have to go to class with hearing kids who were much younger than I. So, I went to work.

Miss Negrini: At the schools in the south and outside of school we used much Ameslan. When I came to California, I found more oral people. I tried to avoid them. The other deaf people in California use lots more good English in their conversations. I found that it required lots of patience to understand them. However, I lived for a while with a girl who had a good command of English, so I learned some from her. I feel that deaf people in California are more socially mature.

Mr. Lowe: My school in Scotland had two separate buildings—one for speech and lipreading only and the other for manual methods. The pupils got together after school. I had no problem in communicating because I could use both methods, but my parents were a problem to me because of their inability to use the English manual alphabet.

Mr. Marquez: I must confess that my conversation with my family is very limited. I am much happier with other deaf people. I have more freedom in talking. I can talk all I want with the deaf.

Mr. Lowe: It is my opinion that deaf people using manual communication are better off in many ways. They go to all places and are happier in many ways.

Mrs. Jacobs: I remember that when I graduated from school and went to the deaf club, I heard about the A.A.A.D. basketball tournaments, the N.A.D., and the Frat. I decided to go to an A.A.A.D. basketball tournament in Kansas City. I went to visit my cousin, who lived there, and went to the basketball games. I sat in an isolated place and watched how happy the deaf people were! The way they greeted each other, hugged their friends, and chatted. I felt so lonely. I was afraid to travel or to go out by myself. One morning a deaf man asked that those who wanted to visit a school for the deaf raise their hands. I raised my hand. I met a deaf girl who was alone, too. We decided to share a hotel room, and we toured the school together. I learned to venture out alone and meet and mix with deaf people. I am now in the group of deaf people who greet each other and hug their friends!

Mr. May: I notice that most of the deaf especially enjoy socializing at sport events such as bowling, basketball games, softball games, etc.

Moderator: How do you get along with hearing people?

Mr. Marquez: Most of my hearing friends warn the others that I can't hear. Then the others try to make me understand them by using speech and gestures.

Miss Negrini: I meet hearing people all the time in bars. They begin to speak to me, then find that I am deaf. They then make things short by using gestures. In order to understand them, I use pencil and pad, facial expressions, or gestures.

Mr. May: When I see hearing people on business, they first ask me if I can lipread them. If not, they then communicate with me with pencil and pad.

Mrs. Burroughs: When I meet hearing people, I can't understand them. I use pencil and pad. At my job I use fingerspelling. I taught some of my co-workers how to fingerspell.

Mr. McCullough: When I was a small boy, the neighborhood kids used homemade signs, gestures, etc., with me. I noticed that when they grew older, they lost interest in me. Very few of them continued to show enough interest in me to use signs and gestures. But, one or two of them went further and learned our language.

Mrs. Jacobs: Many times when you hear or talk well, hearing people begin to expect so much out of you. They think I hear well enough and do not accept the fact of my hearing problem. I am often at a loss to explain my handicap.

Miss Negrini: I can't keep up talking with all the hearing people I meet. I usually find one special person who will go to extra pains to understand and help me. I would rather communicate with her as she is more fun to be with. Sometimes she will influence others to become interested in me.

Moderator: What are your opinions about communication methods?

Mr. Marquez: Not very many hearing people can understand the speech of the deaf unless they can read lip movements.

Mr. May: I think it is better to teach deaf children to communicate manually first and then use total communication later than to have them lipread first. I believe that deaf children should get their education first before learning to lipread.

Mr. McCullough: It is my opinion that all deaf children should learn the total communication method.

Mr. Lowe: It is very difficult to learn speech and lipreading—much more so than the manual method. The school in Scotland places deaf children who can't learn speech in the manual department. The Scottish teachers don't believe in forcing the children to speak and learn lipreading.

Moderator: Can you tell me why so many deaf children are behind hearing children in many ways?

Mrs. Jacobs: I think it is because in most homes no communication exists. For example, deaf children of deaf parents pick up more language skills. I doubt that the participants here had deaf parents. No wonder we had difficulties.

Mr. Marquez: I believe that hearing adults should teach the deaf everything, explain to them how to work by themselves. The deaf are slow because they do not know.

Mr. May: When I entered the Arkansas School, I at first thought I would not be as bright as the other students there because I saw how well they conversed and acted. Then when I went to England, I realized that there were no educational problems for me, and at the Berkeley school I was able to keep up with the others because of my ability in learning new concepts.

Mrs. Burroughs: Many times when my parents talked with each other, I would ask them what they were talking about. And they would always say, "Never mind!" It was hard for me to learn about different things. My parents' friends

looked down at me and made fun of me. I felt bad, but I
could not do anything about it.

Miss Negrini: The deaf are behind in education in general.
They do not do enough reading in school. They play around
too much in school. They go to school just to do the required
work without realizing that education is important. I feel
that teachers should do something to get them to read. When
my hearing friends got to know me better, they realized that
I have a good mind but that I am lazy. They thought I could
read better if I had tried.

Mr. Lowe: I notice that many deaf persons know how to express themselves in signs, but hardly know how to spell
words on paper. And, often they need help with reading,
too.

Mr. McCullough: Deaf teachers get along with and understand deaf children better than hearing teachers. I think that
deaf teachers give the children better lessons, etc.

Moderator: Why do deaf people not mix well with hearing
people?

Miss Negrini: Deaf youngsters stay at residential schools
most of the time, then go out on their own and become
frustrated when they try to get along with other people.
Some succeed, but some don't. The deaf look at hearing
people and feel that they are different. They feel that there is
a barrier between them and the hearing.

Moderator (to Miss Negrini): Why do the deaf feel that they
are different?

Miss Negrini: Just like cats and dogs; they don't get along in
many ways.

Mr. May: I stopped visiting my hearing relatives because
they always left me flat.

Mr. Lowe: I think that hearing people do not come to deaf
people because they are afraid of them—as if they have
smallpox!

Mrs. Jacobs: When I go home to visit my family, Mother
always insists that I visit my many other relatives. I usually

save weekends for my deaf friends, so we have dinners with my relatives on weeknights. Every time my relatives greet me very happily and ask all kinds of questions. Then, five minutes later, they go away by themselves, chatting away. I feel lonely after that and watch TV or read papers. They talk and talk, never bothering to talk with me. I am forgotten!

Mr. May: After leaving Gallaudet College, I met a hearing girl and went with her. I could not keep up with hearing people at parties that she gave; I felt left out. My girl friend felt the same way when she attended parties with deaf people.

Mr. McCullough: I feel that there is a barrier between hearing and deaf people. I believe that some hearing people are "brainwashed" about the deaf. I think hearing people should learn to relate more with the deaf.

Moderator: Why is it that most deaf people usually marry other deaf people? It would seem that if a deaf person were married to a normally hearing person, he could live a much more normal life.

Miss Negrini: Several years ago I went out with a hearing man. I learned very little; our relationship was very limited. I feel that a deaf person should not marry a hearing person. Later, I had a deaf boy friend, and I could see that I could go far and learn a great deal—there was almost no limitation to our relationship.

Mr. May: I did not find the communication I had with my hearing girl friend as good as the communication I had with my ex-wife, who is deaf.

Mrs. Burroughs: My parents wanted me to marry a hearing man, but I married a deaf man, and we are getting along very well.

Mr. Lowe: I told my brother I would much prefer marrying a deaf woman because when I get home late, I would not have to take off my shoes because she would not hear me coming into the house!

Mr. Marquez: During my school days I used to go with a hearing girl. We communicated with pencil and pad. I debated with myself whether to marry her or not. I decided not to. I married a deaf girl. I am much happier. I feel that it would be hard to trust a hearing girl.

Mr. McCullough: Once I went out with two different hearing girls. One could not use manual communication at all, while the other had deaf parents and could talk very well with me. Yet, when we went to gatherings with hearing people, both left me flat to socialize with the other guests. Marriage to a deaf girl would be far more advantageous.

Moderator: Do deaf people really need special service from community service agencies?

Mrs. Jacobs: Yes, because hearing people do not understand the deaf and their varying levels of intelligence. Some of the deaf find it hard to do their best on employment tests. People who know the deaf and their problems can help them get better chances for a good job; they can help the deaf establish better relationships or communication with key hearing persons.

Miss Negrini: I feel that deaf persons should give the special services to other deaf persons. The deaf themselves should become vocational rehabilitation counselors, welfare workers, etc., so that they would be able to understand their clients and their problems.

Mr. May: How can deaf counselors find jobs for their clients without using the telephone?

Miss Negrini: The deaf counselors, etc., can work in their own offices with hearing persons to help with the telephone. The secretaries can make calls for their deaf bosses and write notes when taking calls for them. The counselors can then talk with their deaf clients.

Mrs. Jacobs: When I was looking for a job the last time, I was told by my agency that the boss at the Tribune office felt that since I came from an oral school, I should be able to understand hearing workers and help them relate to deaf workers and vice versa. The boss was not sure of my ability, but the office supervisor knew of a deaf couple who used signs. She was getting along very well with her deaf neighbors. That helped them decide to hire me.

Mr. Marquez: Yes, I think that special services for the deaf are needed. One time I was laid off. My boss asked me how he could get in touch with me when work picked up again. I suggested that he send a telegram to me, and he did so.

Moderator: I have heard that when you lose one sense, like hearing or vision, the other senses become more sensitive and make up for the loss of that sense. What senses do become more sensitive for deaf people?

Mr. May: The sense of sight. I become more visually alert when driving, when associating with hearing people, etc.

Mr. McCullough: We have more extrasensory perception (ESP)!

Mr. Lowe: Many years ago there was some question among the Oregon authorities about allowing the deaf to drive, so a deaf man was prepared for trouble when he went to be examined for his driver's license. The officer asked him what he would do if an emergency vehicle should be coming from behind him. He answered, "When I see the car ahead of me move over, I would move over, too." He got his license to drive.

Miss Negrini: The deaf are usually very observant.

Moderator: Before we finish, I would like you to tell us how you feel about being deaf—are you ashamed or bitter, or are you contented?

Mrs. Jacobs: I am never ashamed of my deafness. I often chat with deaf friends in public places and I sometimes overhear unkind remarks by hearing persons. I speak out to them and that usually makes them feel lousy. I try to educate them about the deaf.

Mr. May: A few times, when hearing people saw me talking on my hands with my deaf friends, they made fun of us by trying to imitate our signs, which hurt my feelings. But, I felt better when I realized that they must be ignorant about deaf people.

Mrs. Jacobs: One day I met a hearing woman waiting for a bus. We just talked. Then, she looked at a blind woman and said, "Poor thing! But, I'd rather be blind than be deaf." I looked at her and said, "Well, I'm deaf but I enjoy looking at things. I do not need to be helped across streets. I look normal in public." The other woman was embarrassed. I told her that music is the only thing that we miss, but that we do feel vibrations.

Mr. May: I am disgusted with hearing persons' using terms like "deaf and dumb" and "deaf mute."

Miss Negrini: I would say that deaf people can be very attractive company, although some hearing persons think that the deaf are stupid. But, more and more hearing people are beginning to understand deafness now.

Mr. Lowe: In Salem, Oregon, one day two deaf men met on the street and began to talk with their hands. A man with a wooden leg came along and watched them. Then he began to ask them questions on paper: "Are you married?" "How many children?" Finally he asked, "Are your children deaf?" The deaf man did not like this question, so he wrote back, "Are you married?" "Yes," was the reply. "Do you have children?" Another "Yes." Then the deaf man asked, "Do they have wooden legs?"

Moderator: This is certainly a good story. I wish to thank all of you for coming and airing your views about deafness. I feel that it was a profitable meeting, because this record of what you think and feel will give the average hearing person a glimpse of what deafness means to a representative group of average deaf adults.

Appendix B

**What Total Family Involvement
Means to Me**

What Total Family Involvement Means to Me

Leo M. Jacobs

(Keynote Speech at International Association of Parents of the Deaf at Gallaudet College, August 8-10, 1975)

I am very much honored to be asked to give the keynote speech to such a nice group of people, for if you subscribe to the philosophy of the IAPD, then you can't be otherwise!

I am sure that you must have heard about "total communication" until it started to come out of your ears, but this philosophy plays a very large part in the concept of total family involvement when a deaf child is concerned.

I believe that you are aware of many unfortunate hearing children who have become unwanted through no fault of their own: Vietnamese children who were disowned and forgotten by their white fathers, foundlings who were left on steps of churches or in restrooms, children of prostitutes or drug addicts, and others. Many of them become disturbed children who grow up into psychopathic adults.

It may be strange to you that I should compare those children with some deaf children who have loving parents—but these deaf children do find themselves in similar situations if their hearing parents possess misdirected goals for their offsprings. These parents fail to realize what deafness means to their children for the handicap is not obvious on the outside surface. Therefore, they persist in wasting their children's precious initial years in attempting to make them poor imitations of hearing children. If they become too absorbed in this hassle with the communicative difficulties of their deaf children, they fail to provide the youngsters with adequate communication tools with which they would have been able to develop intelligence, knowledge, and understanding of their environment. It is saddening to realize that so many loving and concerned parents have, and are still subjecting their deaf children to the same sterile and frustrating experiences that the unwanted hearing children have. These deaf children become disturbed, too, and frequently grow up into adults with psychological problems.

It is simply for this reason that most deaf children of deaf parents do not have the same problems because they do not have any trouble in communicating with their parents. I should know because I had deaf parents. I never even knew that I had a disability until I went to school and began to interact with hearing persons. I was totally involved in my family; I knew everything that my family said and did, and our conversations were interesting and informative. In fact, when I was approaching 12, my mother suggested to my father that he have a good talk with me. So, one evening he asked me to go into the living room with him.

"I think that it is time for us to discuss the facts of life," said my father.

And I said, "All right, Dad. What do you want to know?"

It took me a long time to realize that many of my deaf friends did not have the same full interaction with their families that I had. The full implications did not hit me until I began to work with deaf children, and to find that many of the problems they were facing were unknown to me. But, now, after 37 years of working with deaf youngsters, I am firmly convinced that parents and families make or break their deaf children: their schools can only add to their years of informal education and experiences at home with a modicum of formal academic and vocational training. This is especially true of modern schools for the deaf, which are gradually surrendering their old-time role of surrogate parents due to changing circumstances.

Therefore, it now falls upon today's parents of deaf children to assume a larger and more decisive role with their children. To meet their responsibilities adequately, they must make sure that their youngsters become totally involved with their families. And, to be totally involved with their deaf child and sibling, the hearing members of the family must be one hundred percent proficient in communicating with him. With profoundly deaf children, the need for total communication is undeniable. It is also greatly desirable even with children possessing better hearing.

As I perceive it, a healthy approach toward bringing up deaf children requires that these things should be done: First of all, the parents should accept their deaf child as he is. They should never show by so much as a flicker of expression that they are disappointed in his deafness. They should show their love and delight in their child. They should be as cheerful and positive as possible.

Then, they should communicate with him. They should use *any means* to reach their child and to elicit as full a response as they can from him. They should strive toward a situation where they and their deaf child can exchange thoughts freely and easily. This, then, is when their child will begin his actual education and training.

The natural corollary to the above is to educate him. His parents should tell him about things that he may miss because he can't hear or read. And, they should use positive means to encourage him to read when he becomes ready. They should also teach him values. Although the exemplary approach is the best, the concept of values should always be reinforced through open discussion.

A vital part of raising a child is discipline. Deafness is no excuse for any differential treatment. The parents should treat him/her as they do their other children—the only concession toward their deaf child that they should make is to make sure that the child knows *why* before they act. The kindest thing they can do for the child would be to make him/her realize that he/she will have to take the consequence for behavior which is wrong or unacceptable.

Then, to add some frosting, the parents should foster accomplishments. They should encourage the development of talents and skills which would enhance the child's normal development. The chief reason I am mentioning this item is that these accomplishments would include the acquisition of speech and speechreading skills. These skills should be given prime consideration. You will perhaps note that I am deliberately giving low priority to oral training in the over-all development of the deaf child. This may seem to be heretical to you, but I am convinced that the child will be quicker to pick up oral skills if he/she has first acquired a comprehensive background of knowledge.

These components of the process of rearing a deaf child are effective only if he is an active member of his family, enjoying full exchange of thought with his family. In other words, it is essential that the family be totally involved with the deaf child.

And, this total involvement should produce six-year-old deaf children like Jeffrey, who came downstairs one day, bellowing lustily.

"What's the matter?" asked his mother.

"Papa was hanging pictures, and he just hit his thumb with a hammer," said Jeffrey.

"That's not so serious," soothed his mother. "A big boy like you shouldn't cry at a little thing like that. Why don't you just laugh?"

"I did," sobbed Jeffrey.

I am sure that the parents would have a treasure of such incidents with their deaf children if they would give them a free hand in expressing themselves, and include them as full family members, thus creating a healthy climate for them. In most cases, deaf children are healthy, intelligent, and full of curiosity. What they need is to be given a chance to give full rein to their natural wish to express themselves fully, and to comprehend what is going on outside. Indeed, every household with a deaf child should have tacked on a wall a sign with these words:

EVERY DEAF CHILD HAS THE RIGHT TO UNDERSTAND AND TO BE UNDERSTOOD.

Appendix C

Three Portrayals of Deafness:

Some "Hazards" of Deafness   Roy Holcomb
How Do You Dance Without Music?   Shanny Mow
See! See! See! See! (A Satire)   Lawrence Newman

Some "Hazards" of Deafness

Roy Holcomb

Deafness results in many deviations from everyday living. With care and alertness many of these deviations can be avoided most of the time. However, few deaf people can deny that they have not at one time or another been "victims" of at least a few of the deviations of deafness which follow:("YOU" is the deaf person.)

You start your car but don't feel the vibrations because the motor is running so smoothly. You push the starter again and step on the gas fully. The car makes so much noise that it sounds like a jet getting ready to take off. By-passers give you the "Stupid" look.

While eating at a restaurant the waitress asks you if you care for more coffee. You reply in the negative since your cup is still half full. Later the waitress comes back and says something again. You "catch" only the word "coffee" at the end of her question and reply "yes" assuming that she is repeating her previous question—only this time she has said, "Are you through with your coffee?"

A stranger asks you for a match, directions, or something behind your back or when he does not have your attention. You, of course, do not know it and say nothing. The stranger then gives you a "dirty" look when you do see his face, and you wonder why.

At church the minister asks for all visitors or all those who attend Sunday School, or all those who want to go to hell, or heaven, or some similar question, to stand. You gamble (in church of all places) to stand or sit, knowing that you lose either way.

The doorbell light flashes; you guess the men at the door to be salesmen, since you can't speechread or understand them.

Taking a chance you tell them that you don't care for any. Then the "salesmen" turn out to be delegates from church or charity collectors.

While cleaning the house your vacuum sweeper's cord unintentionally pulled out. You continue to use the vacuum sweeper for several minutes before you realize that it is off. Boy, do you feel dumb!

You take something out of your pocket. Other things come out, too, and fall on the floor without your knowing it. Later, much later, you find yourself missing keys, loose change, or some things which should be in your pockets.

You are in a group of hearing people. You say something not knowing that you have "cut" someone's conversation short.

You pay full admission to movies, night clubs, or other things where sound of one kind or another is part of the price. Then you sit back and "watch" what your money has bought.

You turn around at exactly the right moment, when someone calls you. That person may then scratch his head and wonder if you really are deaf. He may never know that you often look around just to make sure that no one wants you and that all is right with the world.

And how do the deaf accept these "hazards"? Most just laugh at them, pass them along as those you have just read have been passed along. They realize that these deviations are prices which they must pay for their handicap. It would not be wise for them to think in any other way because the acceptance of a handicap and its restricting limitations contributes to a better adjusted individual.

How Do You Dance Without Music?

Shanny Mow

Prologue

My name is Sam. Sometimes I'm called Silent Sam, a tag I loathe out of prejudice—both mine and the bestower's. Besides, it is misleading since I make more noise sipping my soup than the guy at the next table, who is not deaf, but wishes he were every time I take a particularly enthusiastic spoonful.

This is my story, of how I live through a day and the problems I face as a deaf human being, as told to and written by another deaf human being who is fortunate to have the words I do not.

I would be presumptuous to claim that my problems are typical of all deaf persons. Or that I qualify as a Typical Deaf Person, whatever that is. There are the prelingually and post-lingually deaf individuals. There are the college-educated and the illiterate. And those in-between. The hard of hearing. The mentally retarded. The brain damaged. The victims of cerebral palsy. And others. You may say each is a breed apart. Each has problems of his own.

In a style that belies my blue-collar job*, my recorder has set down what I think, what I believe, and what I have gone through.

I can dance better than I can write. Seeing me on the dance floor, hearing people always ask: How do you dance without music? Actually I don't, but I get what they mean. Vibrations, I tell them. Then one night I realized I have been giving an incomplete answer: Now I tell them: Vibrations of life.

"But you can't see a thing from the driver's side," the Volkswagen dealer explains. Sam reads the hurried scribbling

---

*This description of frustrations encountered is applicable for all deaf persons.

and for a minute fingers his new driver's license. Under RESTRICTIONS, it reads LEFT AND RIGHT REAR VIEW MIRRORS.

> Ten dollars goodbye for a right rear view mirror that doesn't give you the view you don't need. Since when did the bureaucrats at the Motor Vehicles decide deafness is a luxury? Be grateful that they let you drive at all?

Wearily he takes the pad and writes, "Install it anyway, I'll be back."

In the noon sun he squints but still can make out the drug store two blocks away. Carefully he looks left, then right and left again, and crosses the street. Midway he pauses to look right again.

> A lot can happen in two blocks. A lost motorist yelling for directions. A nervous smoker asking for a match. A friendly stranger with sinister motives wanting to talk. A policeman blowing his whistle and suspecting you for a fugitive when you walk on. A dog biting from behind. A runaway Safeway cart hitting from the blind side. You grow weary and wary of such people who, at the sight of you pointing to your ear, always seem to forget suddenly their purpose for approaching you. As for whistle-blowing policemen, biting dogs, and runaway carts, you become a staunch believer of oriental fatalism.

Inside the drug store Sam asks for a package of Salem cigarettes, pronouncing the brand name as distinctly as he can. The clerk gives him an odd look, then reaches under the counter. Her hand reappears with the Salems. He breathes easier.

> You feel like a poker player who is also a compulsive bluffer. Mervin Garretson has explained why he switch-

ed brands, rather than fight. As long as you pronounce something safer than Salem, not Chesterfield, there is little danger of receiving cough syrup instead. You can never relax when you cannot hear what you speak. Not even if you've been up to your ears in speech training. Maybe you can, in front of a trained ear, someone who is familiar with the "deaf accent," but unfortunately he is not always around.

Sam also selects a Chapstick and a roll of Lifesavers. The clerk says something which he can at best only guess. His pocket feels heavy with change, but he reaches for his wallet, takes out a dollar bill, and hands it to her.

The tension is even worse when you attempt to lipread. The name of this game is "Figure out the Fingerprint." Like the whorls of his fingertips, each person's lips are different and move in a peculiar way of their own. When young, you build confidence as you guess correctly "ball," "fish," "top," and "shoe" on your teacher's lips. This confidence does not last. As soon as you discover there are more than four words in the dictionary, it evaporates. Seventy percent of the words when appearing on the lips are no more than blurs. Lipreading is a precarious and cruel art which rewards a few who have mastered it and tortures the many who have tried and failed.

The lunch hour is almost over. Sam drives back to the plant, ignoring the new chrome outside his Volkswagen. Several workers nod or wave at him as he makes his way to his workbench. He waves back, but today he feels no desire to join them for the usual noisy banter that precedes the job at hand.

These are good guys. We get along. They like you, even respect you. You laugh at their jokes and fake punches to their jaws. Yet there remains an invisible, insurmountable wall between us. No man can become completely a part of another man's world. He is never more eloquently reminded of this impossibility than when there is no way he can talk with the other man.

Without a word, the foreman nods. Sam scribbles down another question. The foreman nods again. Still another question. More nodding, this time with marked annoyance. Sam then knows it is pointless to continue.

Communication is the father of human relationships. From infancy a person learns to speak at a rate closely synchronized with his thinking processes. Deviation from this timing between thinking and speaking upsets his natural flow of thought. He loses his tongue or forces out words which sound so artificial that they disgust him. As a deaf person, you sympathize with this mental block in the hearing person who tries to speak to you. In fact, you expect it. For this reason, just or not, you always wonder why he takes the trouble to speak to you.

You feel no less helpless in your search for meaningful communication. When the hearing person does not know, as he usually does not, the sign language, the only recourse lies with the pencil and pad. Here your language defeats you before you begin. You have been deprived of the natural process of learning language, i.e., by the ear. You do not start from scratch when you begin your formal education. The itch is not even there. English is a language so complicated and inconsistent that its mastery is for you as elusive as the pot of gold at the end of the rainbow. Gamely you pick up the pencil only to find the hearing person hung-up in his own way: poor penmanship, bad spelling, or some other reason known only to him. Inhibition reduces communication to a superficial level, a most unsatisfactory relationship to both parties. Speech and lipreading? Try discussing

Kazantzakis, or any subject, limiting yourself to the 30 percent of the words that can be lipread with no guarantee that there would be none of the words you have not seen before.

Tired as he is, Sam cannot go home yet. He remembers he has a couple of errands to perform. He surveys the traffic. It is getting bad. He tries but cannot think of a short cut to the other side of town where Paul lives. He shifts the gears, passing one roadside booth after another, each displaying the familiar Bell symbol.

His finger is tiring. From pressing continuously the door button that is rigged to a light bulb inside. He searches through a window, then another. No sign of life except for the parakeet. Refraining from kicking the door, he hastily writes down the message, inserts it in a crack in the door and returns to his car. Sweat streaks down his forehead, and he wipes it away. Hopefully he eyes the door once more.

How soon will you get Paul's reply? Will the note still be there when he comes home? When will he come home? He could not know you were driving down. You took your chance and lost. An alternate to this eternal courtship with chance is to plan ahead. Carry out, no wavering. Build a reputation of a man of his word. Your word determines the kind of relationship you will enjoy with your fellowmen. It does not have the freedom and flexibility made possible by the telephone with its sanctuary of distance, so dear to the hearing person at the eleventh hour. When you have committed yourself, by mail or in a previous visit, to come to a party, you come. Even if you are feeling particularly misanthropic that night. You may excuse yourself with a few days' advance notice, again by mail or in person, but you have to be mighty convincing when you explain to the host that Jeanne Dixon has divulged the future to you—that on the night of the party you would feel terribly anti-social, therefore it would be wise if you stay away.

"Your number is 48," the girl behind the counter smiles sweetly and turns to the next customer. Sam hesitates, then shrugs and finds a seat close to the TAKE-OUT counter.

Bright kid, this girl. She reacted as if there is nothing out of the ordinary when a customer grabs the order pad and places his own order. No doubt she is also a great believer of miracles, that somehow your deafness will disappear before your pizza is ready and the number, whatever it is, announced on the loudspeaker.

The pizza tastes cold but good. Sam settles back and watches with affection as Brian and Brenda finish their portions. He waits until Jane returns with the coffee before waving for the family's attention. "Want to go to the lake next week?" he more announces than asks with his hands and fingers. Shrieks of delight answer him, unheard.

In group discussions where you alone are deaf, you do not exist. Because you cannot present your ideas through a medium everyone is accustomed to, you are not expected, much less asked, to contribute them. Because you are deaf, they turn deaf. Just do what your parents, friends, fellow workers—who can hear—tell you; you will know soon enough as we go along. Yours is not to reason why; yours is to do and die silently. Does no one realize that security comes from knowing what you will be doing next, knowing what to expect? Does no one agree that much of the joy of performing an activity stems from the realization that you had a hand in planning it?

"Yes, you may bring Barb and Jo along," Sam smiles as Brenda hugs the dolls and skips happily out of the room. To his seven-year-old son, he asks, "Brian, tell me, what can we do at the lake?"

You never forget that frightening experience. When you were Brian's age, you were left out of the dinner table conversation. It is called mental isolation. While everyone is talking or laughing, you are as far away as a lone Arab on a desert that stretches along every horizon. Everyone and everything are a mirage; you see them but you cannot touch or become a part of them. You thirst for connection. You suffocate inside but you cannot tell anyone of this horrible feeling. You do not know how to. You get the impression nobody understands or cares. You have no one to share your childish enthusiasm and curiosity, no sympathetic listener who can give meaning to your world and the desert around you. You are not granted even the illusion of participation. You are expected to spend 15 years in the straitjacket of speech training and lipreading. You learn not how to communicate, only how to parrot words, never to speak your own. Meantime your parents never bother to put in an hour a day to learn sign language or some part of it. One hour out of 24 that can change a lifetime for you. Instead, the most natural form of expression for you is dismissed as vulgar. It has never occurred to them that communication is more than method or talk. That it is a sense of belonging, an exchange of understanding, a mutual respect for the other's humanity.

The kids have been put in bed, Sam pours a third cup of coffee for himself. Jane is doing the dishes, and he decides to get his pipe from the living room. He cannot find it and returns to the kitchen.

Your eyes are your contact with the world, but there is only so much you can see. Seeing is waiting. From the living room you cannot ask Jane about the pipe. In the kitchen you cannot ask while she is washing the carving knife. She cannot answer until the knife is safely put down. You must stop with half of the shaving lather still on your face to answer how you want your eggs done. Then Jane must hurry back to the kitchen before the waffle burns. You always have laryngitis when you call Brian and Brenda to supper. It is rude to notice the fly in your pie while Jane is talking. You must walk across the room and touch her shoulder if you want her attention. Or stamp on the floor and probably ruin her mood or concentration for the next half hour.

He almost spills the coffee. "Sorry, honey," Jane smiles.

"Did Bill come to the plant to see you?" she asks. Sam nods and adds, "And he was sore like a wounded bear." He takes two cubes of sugar and stirs the coffee. He puts the spoon down. "It's about the latest federal grant for a project on some problems of the deaf, " he explains. "Exactly what problems, I don't know. Bill isn't sure either, but he does know who is going to head it."

It is always someone with the magic prefix "Dr." before his name or some connection with some prestigious but distant institution. Someone Bill has run across at a recent workshop and asked:

"Have you had any practical experience, say teaching, in the field of 'deaf education'?"

"No."

"Have you had any professional connection with a residential school for the deaf or some large day class for the deaf?"

"No."

"Do you know a deaf person personally?"

"No."

"In your professional capacity, have you ever worked with a deaf person, this person being either an associate or subordinate?"

"No."

"Have you ever been to a club for the deaf or some social gathering of the deaf?"

"No."

"Do you socialize with the deaf?"

"No."

"Have you ever spent a night in a discussion or chat with a deaf person?"

"No."

"In this workshop, do you integrate with deaf participants during the coffee breaks?"

"No."

"Did you try to?"

"No."

"Do you know how to communicate manually?"

"No."

"Do you believe the child should have a choice in methods of communication for the greatest stimulation of his intellectual growth?"

"No."

"One more question, sir. Would you attribute our failures in educating and rehabilitating the deaf to a lack of understanding of the subject and its problems?"

"Yes. It's a damned shame. Let me tell you about this research I'm . . ."

Yes, it's a damned shame. Thanks to these armchair academicians, you find yourself cynical or apathetic toward the projects and programs that have been set up to improve your lot, including those run by other professional people in the field, who are more open and honest, who have so rubbed elbows with you that their elbows ache if they do not move in a conversation with you. You are an American Indian resenting the white hearing man far away in some ivy-covered Indian Bureau, who has never laid his eyes on you but feels himself nevertheless qualified to declare what is wrong with you and to dictate your destiny.

Or you are too preoccupied in your struggle for a happy and meaningful life to give a hoot about these projects and programs. More than the hearing person, you need all the extra time you can get to achieve any ambitious goal. Yet you are expected by your own kind, by the "deaf intellectuals" to sacrifice this extra time to the cause of the deaf image, to help your less fortunate deaf brothers. You may even be expected to change jobs for one in which you can carry a larger part in this holy mission. You are under constant pressure to behave only in a manner favorable to this image.

The man on the tube looks as if he has a goldfish flipping inside his mouth. He refuses to leave; another joins him, mouthing likewise. Sam sighs and reaches for the channel dial. In a split second the Shakespeare Special is replaced by an undersea scene.

A big fish approaches the diver. Barracuda? It is going to attack the diver, or is it? Why does it hesitate, then swim off? What did the diver do that was not visibly obvious? Would he have been attacked had he acted otherwise? But is the damn fish some kind of shark? The commentator supplies all the answers, but they pass through you as if you were a sieve. Desperately you grab for what you can, but you cannot see what you cannot hear. A wealth of information, both practical and exotic, escapes you daily. Television, movies, and the stage hold limited meaning for you. Radio, phonograph players, tape recorders, and loud speakers have none. Then to what do you turn for information? The nearby human being is too unreliable. So you have only books. Read twice, thrice, four times as much as the average person to know just as much. Slowly you close the cultural gap that is widening even faster by the incredible speed and ease of modern media.

Sam is alone in the living room, illuminated by a single lamp. Jane has long since retired, but he himself feels no urgency for sleep. From the coffee table he picks up Remarque's *All Quiet on the Western Front.* Hardly has he opened the book before he reaches for the dictionary.

What are haricot beans? Mess-tin? Dollop? Voracity? Already four words out of your vocabulary, all from the first paragraph on the first page! You read this classic as an adult while other read it in their teens. You are lucky you can recognize the words as English. For some deaf adults they might as well be trying to read the original version in German. Others with a little more reading ability plod through page by page, their laborious effort dimming the brilliant power of the message and the brutal grace of the story. In addition, there are unfamiliar idioms, colloquialisms, and expressions. The difficult language which you have never mastered makes for difficult reading. As if it is not enough, you often lack the background information necessary for comprehension of the subject. Scratch out another—or your last—reliable source of information.

Finishing a chapter, he puts the book down and closes the edgeworn dictionary. He rubs his eyes and stretches his arms. The *Tribune* comes in his field of vision and he opens it to the classified ads section.

Maybe there's something you overlooked earlier tonight . . . Yes, here's a possibility . . . Damn it, no address, just a lousy phone number . . . Have you had enough of the job at the plant? Eight years of brain-numbing drudgery. Is one such a coward not to quit? When you contemplate a job change, you are not as half concerned about the new location, working conditions, fringe benefits, school for your children, new friends, etc., as you are about basic survival and a decent income that will permit your family to live in relative comfort. You don't move on because you itch for a change of scenery or because your boss doesn't like the length of your hair. You do not doubt your ability to change jobs, to perform the job or to keep the job, only whether you would be given a chance to prove this ability, to convince the prospective but skeptical employer that ability is all that counts. You can't write or read well. You can't speak. How do you sell yourself, by drawing pictures? All things being equal, the job goes to the applicant whose ears do not just hold up his eyeglasses.

Against the vast black nothingness, a fleck of light winks here and there, like distant planets greeting a lost traveler. Watching through the window, Sam suddenly realizes how much he loves the city.

In one city you dare not hope for many job openings, any kind, where the deafness of a worker is treated as irrelevant or routine. You may have to cross a dozen city limits, perhaps half a continent, before you find one. Then the lesser factors take on new importance, such as the slow and often painful acceptance of Brian and Brenda by their new playmates. The children are still learning to live with their and your handicap. Then there is the search for housing in want ads which seem to conspire against you, listing only phone numbers for the most desirable and reasonably-priced units. And the orientation of local merchants and new neighbors to your deafness. And the deaf population in the new city which may turn out to consist entirely of your family. You are well settled here. Need you push your luck?

Slowly he folds the paper and gets up. He switches the lamp

off and walks cautiously down the dark hall. His hands move along the wall, keeping in contact for balance because his balance was affected when he became deaf. At the door of his bedroom he pauses. As his eyes adjust to the darkness, he can make out the features of Jane's face.

Sam, do you love her or are you merely fond of her? You married her because she was available, the best of a limited lot. Probably she had said "Yes" for the same reason. It has always been this way: You don't have a ghost of a choice about your own education, ambition, job, wife, friends, recreation, and sometimes religion. For you, choice is a limited word. You are the novelist's delight, the lonely, soul-searching character who has never found what he seeks in life. Unlike the perennial wanderer, you know which road you want to travel, but you keep running into one roadblock or another. The day you lost you hearing your universe shrank many times over; your power of choice in a world of sound became drastically reduced. Thrown in the storm of silence, you seek refuge among your own kind and become part of a microcosm which you are not sure you want. It is a closed society whose bond among members is founded not on mutual interests or intellectual equality but on a common desire for escape from the "cruel outside world," for communication, although this communication frequently turns out to be an illusion. It breeds dependence, stagnation, pettiness, and finally boredom. It is a microcosm that unmercifully tries your individuality. You either surrender to tribal conformity or return to the other world. Or live on the fringes of both worlds, never to fully accept one and never to be fully accepted by the other.

He tosses in the bed. Unable to sleep, he stares at the far corner of the room. Jane stirs but is still again. He moves his hands to the back of his head and folds them.

Are you indulging in excessive self-pity? Brood and brood until there is no objectivity left in you? Is that why psychologists analyze you as being self-centered, immature, suspicious and narrow-minded, always self-conscious, and defensive about your inability to hear? An unhealthy mental attitude? Or shall we call it inevitable? This outlook is not a product of deafness per se but of the general public attitude, or ignorance, to the nature of deafness and the problems it creates.

Imagine yourself in a living room full of people who all know what is going on. Except you, who inquires and is answered with a polite smile which only underlines your helplessness. Everyone seems relaxed, enjoying himself. Except you, who is uneasily waiting for something to happen which makes sense to you. Everyone chats congenially with one another. Except you, who receives more polite smiles and fugitive glances. Everyone tells something hilarious and laughs. Except you, who debates with yourself whether you would appear less ridiculous going along and laughing at Godknowswhat or remaining stoic thus making your deafness even more conspicuous in an atmosphere already made uneasy by your presence.

Leaving the room means crawling back into your "deaf shell" from which you seek escape in the first place. A triumph of futility. So you stay on, making the best of your dilemma, waiting, hoping for the breakthrough when someone will realize you are indeed human. And tolerance may yet become acceptance.

You find it difficult to forget for a moment you are deaf when you are continuously reminded by an unwitting public. You are daily subjected to this public's unpredictable reaction and to the necessity of proving yourself. A lifetime of unending strain. After all this, can you kid yourself about not becoming oversensitive in your human relationships?

You know you are getting a raw deal but you do not know whom to blame. Public ignorance is a faceless enemy against whom you cannot fight with force. How do you get a society to accept you when it is ruled by this enemy? It can be educated to show understanding, compassion, but it does not always listen. Sometimes you wonder why it seems to be afraid of you.

People are however not your *raison d'etre*. Each unpleasant episode with them is an unavoidable skirmish. They represent only obstacles in your battle. The objective of the battle is a life in which you can sing between dejections, laugh between tears, dream between nightmares, breathe between repressions, love between prejudices, and grow between defeats. And, by God, you are making it.

Peace settles over Sam. He falls asleep with his arms around Jane.

See! See! See! See!

Lawrence Newman

In medical terms John had what was called *ophthalmia neonatorum,* an eye infection which left him with ten percent vision, mostly in the right eye. The first time John went to school, he was amazed to learn that the use of braille was not only frowned upon but strictly forbidden. "You see," the school people told him, "braille becomes a crutch and will prevent you from using what residual seeing you have. By leaning on braille you will be following the line of least resistance."

Words were a blur even when a magazine was held close to his eyes, but John did not complain. He had faith in his school officials. Did they not have a lot of experience? And the years they spent in college . . . What's more, their statements sounded so logical, such as the following: "This is a seeing world, the kind in which you will have to live. Do seeing people use braille?" There was even a motto in the principal's office: "SEE! SEE! SEE! SEE!"

John's parents were firmly behind the school. Yes, they were 100 percent behind the school because they wanted John to be as normal as possible. Constant exposure to the world of sight, they learned, was important. They even had special eyeglasses fitted for their son to help increase the acuity of his remnant sight and to make his drooping eyelids less conspicuous. The school taught him how to lift his drooping eyelids so that he could appear as normal as possible.

No one could say that John did not try. He eventually could make out large letters in newspaper headlines. His parents were excited and pleased when he showed them what he could do. The school officials were in a dither with John's achievement. They called in the newspapers, and soon John's story was carried by the wire services throughout the nation. The school took John on many trips to demonstrate his ability. He performed before the Daughters of ----, the Charity of ----, the Auxiliary Sisters of ----, to mention but three. Many were moved to tears, and some even hugged and kissed John.

Soon something was troubling John. Some of his schoolmates were smuggling in magazines and books in braille although these were not permitted even outside the classroom. His schoolmates surreptitiously urged John to learn braille. He refused to be contaminated even though some of the arguments of his classmates carried a more logical ring than those of the school people. One congenitally blind boy told him he had no vision so what was he supposed to do? John was flabbergasted because he had been told that every blind person had some residual vision, no matter how little, that could be utilized. The same boy said that if a flashlight was stuck to his eye, he could sense some light but what good would that do?

Another girl, an acquired blindness case, said that she had some vision left, a very small percent, but that after ten years she still could not tell the letters ''m'' and ''n'' apart; sometimes the tail of the ''j'' appeared faded and therefore looked like an ''i''; and the ''o'' sometimes became a ''p''. With a sigh she mentioned that time was when she could tell a boy and a girl apart in the distance, but not any more.

What shocked John more than anything else was the news via the grapevine to the effect that almost all blind persons use braille. Braille? Almost all? He began to waver when he learned that there were some schools where braille was permitted outside of the classroom. He was staggered even further to know that there were schools that even permitted braille in the classroom!

John slowly began to realize how surface appearances could be deceptive. There is a form of eye trouble called *conjunctivitis,* and those who have this are not really blind but only hard-of-seeing. This type of student—along with those who acquired blindness late in life and could therefore remember many sights and objects and their shape, texture, and color—was often used to demonstrate the success of a school's method. The school's policy and methodology were geared for the benefit of these types. They were often portrayed on television and featured in the press—and the public was misled. Those not in the know or who were fed the one-and-only method looked askance at those who used braille or could not use their seeing skills: such unfortunates were considered primitive or backward or just plain dumb!

John began to ask himself what good it was to be able to read large headlines if he could not read without facility and understanding whole columns which were the "meat" of what the headlines were screaming. He began to ask himself what it really meant to live in a seeing world.

Which is more important, John kept asking himself: to assume an appearance of normalcy with 10% vision that stumbles and staggers, OR to admit having a sight impairment, letting the world know it, and using braille to advance and ensure his place in that world. Which? Which?

"Hey, Bill!" he called out to one of his classmates, "Take my hand and show me what all these dots mean." John felt a sense of elation as Bill guided him. "Yes, yes, this is 'A'—and what?"

"'A' stands for 'Alice' . . ."*

---

*Alice Cogswell, the first deaf girl taught the manual alphabet by Thomas Hopkins Gallaudet.

Index

This book was typeset in phototype Baskerville by Litho Comp, Inc. of Bethesda, Maryland. It was printed and bound by Bookcrafters, Inc. of Chelsea, Michigan. The book and jacket were designed by Donna Simons.